P9-AOX-593

The Trained Mind

Total Concentration

Fitness, Health & Nutrition was created by Rebus, Inc. and published by Time-Life Books.

REBUS, INC.

Publisher: RODNEY FRIEDMAN
Editorial Director: CHARLES L. MEE JR.

Editor: THOMAS DICKEY
Senior Editor: WILLIAM DUNNETT
Text Editor: LINDA EPSTEIN
Associate Editors: MARY CROWLEY, CARL LOWE
Chief of Research: CARNEY W. MIMMS III
Assistant Editor: PENELOPE CLARK
Copy Editor: ROBERT HERNANDEZ
Contributing Editor: JACQUELINE DAMIAN

Art Director: JUDITH HENRY
Associate Art Director: FRANCINE KASS
Designer: SARA BOWMAN
Still Life and Food Photographer: STEVEN MAYS
Exercise Photographer: ANDREW ECCLES
Photo Stylists: LINDSAY DIMEO, LEAH LOCOCO
Photo Assistant: TIMOTHY JEFFS

Test Kitchen Director: GRACE YOUNG
Recipe Editor: BONNIE J. SLOTNICK

Time-Life Books Inc. is a wholly owned subsidiary of

TIME INCORPORATED

Founder: HENRY R. LUCE 1898-1967

Editor-in-Chief: JASON MCMANUS
Chairman and Chief Executive Officer: J. RICHARD MUNRO
President and Chief Operating Officer: N.J. NICHOLAS JR.
Corporate Editor: RAY CAVE
Executive Vice President, Books: KELSO F. SUTTON
Vice President, Books: GEORGE ARTANDI

TIME-LIFE BOOKS INC.

Editor: GEORGE CONSTABLE

Executive Editor: ELLEN PHILLIPS
Director of Design: LOUIS KLEIN
Director of Editorial Resources: PHYLLIS K. WISE
Editorial Board: RUSSELL B. ADAMS JR., DALE M. BROWN, ROBERTA CONLAN, THOMAS H. FLAHERTY, LEE HASSIG, DONIA ANN STEELE, ROSALIND STUBENBERG, HENRY WOODHEAD
Director of Photography and Research: JOHN CONRAD WEISER
Assistant Director of Editorial Resources: ELISE RITTER GIBSON

President: CHRISTOPHER T. LINEN
Chief Operating Officer: JOHN M. FAHEY JR.
Senior Vice Presidents: ROBERT M. DESENA, JAMES L. MERCER, PAUL R. STEWART
Vice Presidents: STEPHEN L. BAIR, RALPH J. CUOMO, NEAL GOFF, STEPHEN L. GOLDSTEIN, JUANITA T. JAMES, HALLETT JOHNSON III, CAROL KAPLAN, SUSAN J. MARUYAMA, ROBERT H. SMITH, JOSEPH J. WARD
Director of Production Services: ROBERT J. PASSANTINO

EDITORIAL BOARD OF ADVISORS

Peter Apor, M.D., Ph.D., Director, Department of Fitness and Recreation, Szabadsaghegyi Children's Hospital, Budapest, Hungary

Eva S. Auchincloss, Consultant, Women's Sports Foundation

Dorothy V. Harris, Ph.D., Professor, Laboratory for Human Performance Research, The Pennsylvania State University; U.S. Olympic Sports Psychology Advisory Committee

Hans Howald, M.D., Professor, Biochemistry of Exercise, Swiss National Training Institute, Magglingen, Switzerland

Paavo V. Komi, Ph.D., Professor, Department of Biology of Physical Activity, University of Jyvaskyla, Finland

Joyce C. Lashof, M.D., Dean, School of Public Health, University of California, Berkeley

Joyce T. Leung, R.D., M.S., M.P.H., Department of Pediatrics, Columbia University

William D. McArdle, Ph.D., Professor, Department of Health and Physical Education, Queens College

Sheldon Margen, M.D., Professor, Department of Public Health Nutrition, University of California, Berkeley

Jeffrey Minkoff, M.D., Director, Sports Medicine Center, New York University

Mitsumasa Miyashita, Ph.D., Professor, Laboratory for Exercise Physiology and Biomechanics, Tokyo University, Japan; Fellow, American College of Sports Medicine

Richard C. Nelson, Ph.D., Director, Biomechanics Laboratory, The Pennsylvania State University

Benno M. Nigg, Ph.D., Director, Laboratory for Human Performance Studies, Faculty of Physical Education, University of Calgary, Canada

Ralph S. Paffenbarger Jr., M.D., Professor of Epidemiology, Department of Family, Community and Preventive Medicine, Stanford University School of Medicine

Jana Parizkova, M.D., Ph.D., D.Sc., Professor, Research Institute for Physical Education, Charles University, Prague, Czechoslovakia

V.A. Rogozkin, Professor, Research Institute of Physical Culture, Leningrad, U.S.S.R.

Allan J. Ryan, M.D., Director, Sports Medicine Enterprise; former Editor-in-Chief, *The Physician and Sportsmedicine*

Bengt Saltin, M.D., Ph.D., Professor, August Krogh Institute, University of Copenhagen, Denmark

Christine L. Wells, Ph.D., Professor, Department of Health and Physical Education, Arizona State University

Myron Winick, M.D., R.R. Williams Professor of Nutrition, Institute of Human Nutrition, College of Physicians and Surgeons, Columbia University

William B. Zuti, Ph.D., Director, Pepsico Fitness Center; Fellow, American College of Sports Medicine; former national director of health enhancement, YMCA

FITNESS, HEALTH & NUTRITION

The Trained Mind

Total Concentration

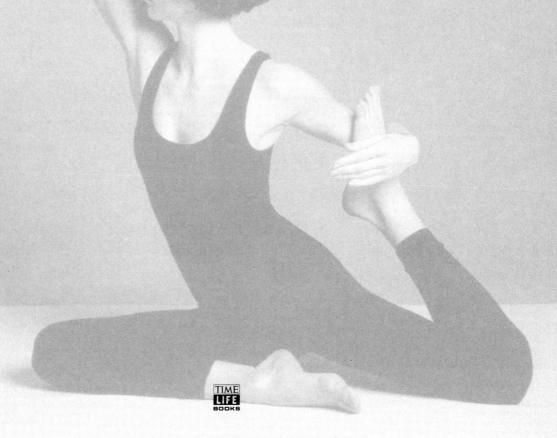

Time-Life Books, Alexandria, Virginia

CONSULTANTS FOR THIS BOOK

Rod K. Dishman, Ph.D., is Associate Professor and Director of the Behavioral Fitness Laboratory at the University of Georgia, Athens. He serves on numerous committees, including the executive committee of the Division of Exercise and Sports Psychology of the American Psychological Association, and the Sports Medicine Council of the United States Olympic Committee. In addition, he is an Associate Editor of *Medicine and Science in Sports and Exercise* and is on the editorial board of the *Journal of Sports Psychology.*

Dorothy V. Harris, Ph.D., is Professor of Exercise and Sports Science at Pennsylvania State University and Education Director of the Women's Sports Foundation in New York. As the first sports psychologist in residence at the Olympic Training Center in Colorado Springs, she has worked with many elite athletes. She is the author of *The Athlete's Guide to Sports Psychology: Mental Skills for Physical People.*

Charlotte Honda is a Certified Movement Analyst and an Associate Professor in Health and Physical Education at Bronx Community College in New York. She has 20 years of experience teaching Hatha Yoga, dance and movement.

Scott Pengelly, Ph.D., is a sports psychologist for Nike and for Athletics West, an elite track and field team. Dr. Pengelly has consulted with athletes in both professional and amateur sports, helping them compete in national and international championships, including the Olympics.

Henry Smith is a martial arts instructor who holds a 4th-degree black belt in Aikido and a 2nd-degree black belt in Iaido, the Samurai art of swordsmanship. An experienced dancer and choreographer as well as a teacher, he is the artistic director of Solaris Dance Theatre in New York City and the creator of the Warrioraerobics Fitness Program, which he teaches internationally.

Nutritional consultants:

Ann Grandjean, Ed.D., is Associate Director of the Swanson Center for Nutrition, Omaha, Neb.; chief nutrition consultant to the U.S. Olympic Committee; and an instructor in the Sports Medicine Program, Orthopedic Surgery Department, University of Nebraska Medical Center.

Myron Winick, M.D., is the R.R. Williams Professor of Nutrition, Professor of Pediatrics, Director of the Institute of Human Nutrition, and Director of the Center for Nutrition, Genetics and Human Development at Columbia University College of Physicians and Surgeons. He has served on the Food and Nutrition Board of the National Academy of Sciences and is the author of many books, including *Your Personalized Health Profile.*

For information about any Time-Life book please call 1-800-621-7026, or write:
Reader Information
Time-Life Customer Service
P.O. Box C-32068
Richmond, Virginia 23261-2068

©1988 Time-Life Books Inc. All rights reserved. No part of this book may be reproduced in any form or by any electronic or mechanical means, including information storage and retrieval devices or systems, without prior written permission from the publisher except that brief passages may be quoted for reviews. First printing.

Published simultaneously in Canada.
School and library distribution by Silver Burdett Company, Morristown, New Jersey.

TIME-LIFE is a trademark of Time Incorporated U.S.A.

Library of Congress Cataloging-in-Publication Data
The Trained mind: total concentration.
    p. cm. — (Fitness, health & nutrition)
Includes index.
    ISBN 0-8094-6118-8
    ISBN 0-8094-6119-6 (lib. bdg.)
    1. Stress (Psychology) — Prevention.
2. Yoga, Hatha — Therapeutic use.
3. Meditation — Therapeutic use.
4. Relaxation — Therapeutic use. 5. Mind and body. I. Time-Life Books. II. Series: Fitness, health, and nutrition.
RC455.4.S87T73 1988
613 — dc 19   88-19182
                      CIP

This book is not intended as a substitute for the advice of a physician. Readers who have or suspect they may have specific medical problems should consult a physician about any suggestions made in this book. Readers beginning a program of rehabilitative or strenuous physical exercise are also urged to consult a physician.

CONTENTS

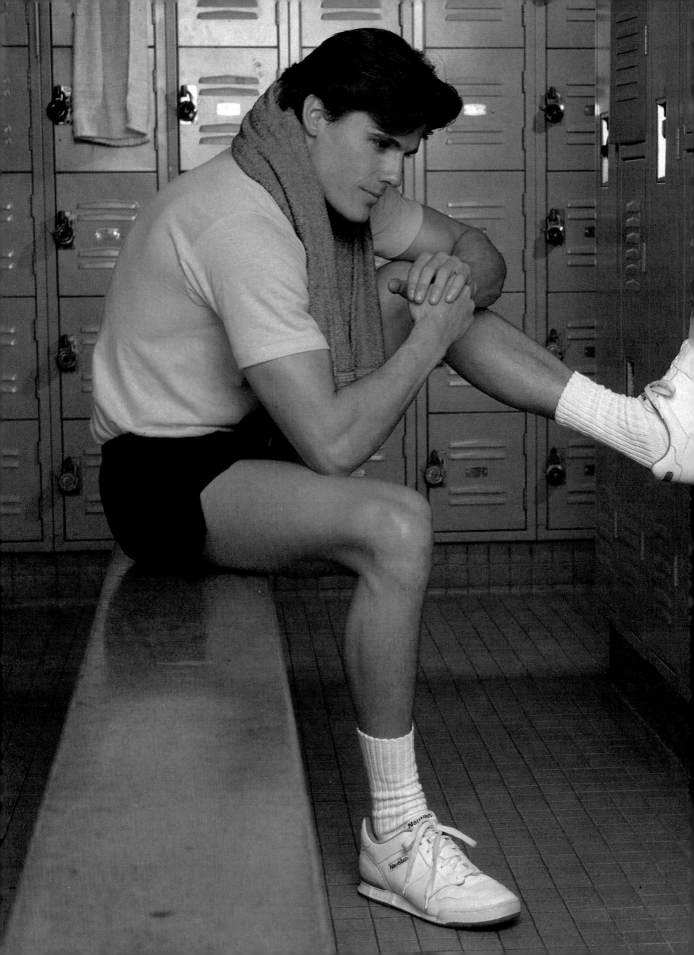

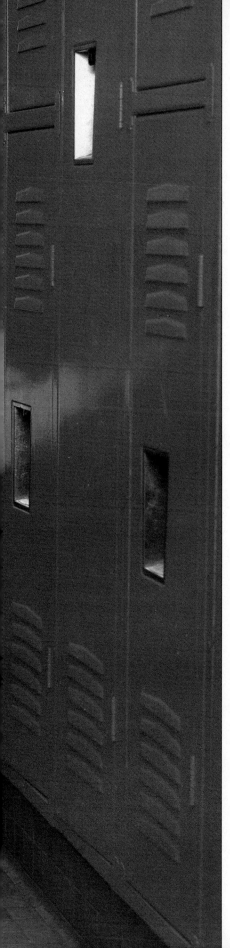

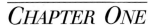
The Mind and Performance

*How mental training can help
you function at your best*

As researchers learn more about the human body's performance capabilities, there is increasing evidence that a person's physical state can be affected substantially by his or her mental state. Studies have shown that it is possible voluntarily to control such unconscious autonomic functions as heart rate, skin temperature and muscle tension, as well as many emotional reactions to stress. Many athletes claim that the mental aspect of training and competing is crucial to how well they perform. Yet until recently, athletes and coaches frequently believed that such skills as the ability to relax and concentrate are simply personality traits. This chapter explains how and why these skills, in fact, can be learned and improved. The techniques for accomplishing this, which are covered in subsequent chapters, can not only raise physical performance to higher levels of excellence, but can also make any game, workout or training regimen more enjoyable and productive.

What goes through runners' minds during a marathon? Some runners use what researchers call dissociative thinking to take their minds off the race — thoughts about chocolate cake or the post-race party, for example. Others use an associative strategy, paying close attention to their bodily functions — respiration, stride, arm swing and others. The top finishers are among the associative group: Both elite athletes and amateur runners who use associative thinking finish faster than runners who let their minds wander.

What is mental training?

This is a general phrase for strategies, techniques and exercises based on a fundamental principle of sports psychology — that psychological skills can be developed in much the same way that physical skills are. Although it is true that we have certain innate traits and limitations, it is well established that most people can train their bodies to perform a physical activity better through exercise and practice. In recent years, several sports psychologists have demonstrated that the same is true of mental capabilities. More and more, their research has established that the ability to concentrate, to relax under pressure, to feel more confident and motivated can all be enhanced through exercises specifically aimed at accomplishing these improvements.

Some conditioning methods are strictly mental, while others require particular body motions and positions to achieve a psychological response. Both methods have been successful enough that many athletes now seek out the assistance of sports psychologists. Recently the United States Olympic Committee acknowledged the importance of sports psychology and is sponsoring training programs for many of the Olympic athletes.

What can training your mind accomplish?

Whether you work out in a gym, play a skilled game like tennis or train and compete in an endurance activity like a marathon, you may not perform well consistently. There are days when everything feels right — when muscles are loose, energy is flowing and responses are sharp. Then there are days when your performance is off — you cannot lift the same amount of weight you did two days before; on a tennis court, you keep missing shots and lose to a less-talented opponent; you simply run out of stamina and mental energy and drop out of a race without finishing.

This day-to-day performance fluctuation is not attributable necessarily to shifts in physical skills and conditioning: It is the mind that fails to perform well consistently. This is most evident in top athletes who are on a par physically and recognize that their mental attitude can be 90 percent responsible for the outcome of an event. However, the mind's role is important for people at all skill levels in every situation. Whenever you feel you should have performed better or if you are not enjoying a game — during exercise or in competition — you must consider your state of mind.

What mental attributes will help you perform well?

From information reported by athletes, sports psychologists have identified several factors that contribute to excellent performance. When they compete, many athletes are aware of having a high degree of concentration, of being extraordinarily focused on the task at hand. In this focused state, they feel no need to exert control over their situation; they have a sense of effortlessly being in charge of themselves and of the game. They are not consciously aware of every little

Balancing Act: Controlling the Stress State

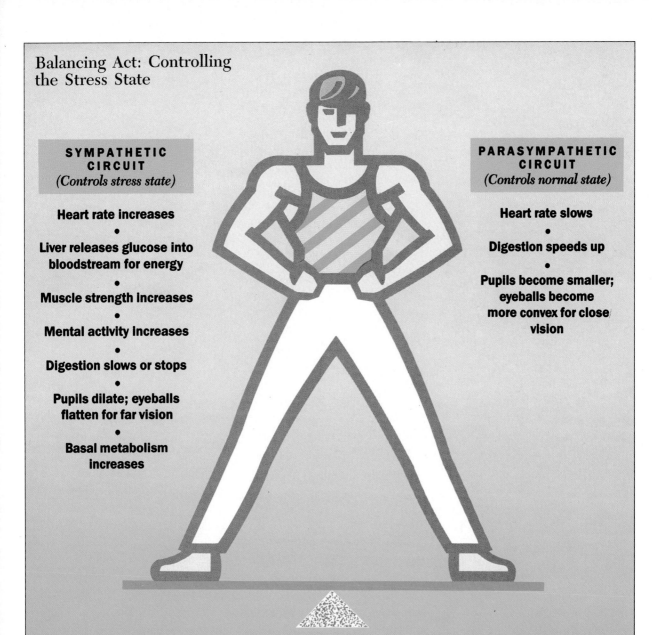

SYMPATHETIC CIRCUIT
(Controls stress state)

Heart rate increases

•

Liver releases glucose into bloodstream for energy

•

Muscle strength increases

•

Mental activity increases

•

Digestion slows or stops

•

Pupils dilate; eyeballs flatten for far vision

•

Basal metabolism increases

PARASYMPATHETIC CIRCUIT
(Controls normal state)

Heart rate slows

•

Digestion speeds up

•

Pupils become smaller; eyeballs become more convex for close vision

Vigorous physical activity, like certain emotional circumstances, produces an aroused, or stressful, state that is accompanied by a number of specific physiological changes. These changes are linked to the body's autonomic nervous system, which governs such functions as heart rate, sweating and digestion. The autonomic nervous system adjusts these functions continually in order to meet the changing environment.

As shown above, the autonomic nervous system is actually composed of two separate systems, or circuits: the sympathetic and the parasympathetic. It is these systems that regulate the body's reponses to stress. During calm, balanced emotional states, the parasympathetic system controls automatic bodily functions. Under stress, the sympathetic system comes into play, preparing your body to meet the challenge by increasing your heart rate, respiration, muscular tension and nutrient energy supply. These sympathetic changes, which together are known as the "fight or flight" response, occur rapidly and are normal, necessary elements of reaching an optimal level of arousal for peak performance. But the sympathetic circuit must be controlled, otherwise stress turns into anxiety and your performance will deteriorate. Such activities as meditation, Yoga, self-talk, progressive relaxation and visualization work to engage the parasympathetic circuit again in order to balance the body's two automatic circuits.

The Four Types of Attention

Attention has two dimensions: width (broad or narrow) and direction (internal or external). The interplay of these dimensions results in four basic types of attention *(right),* among which you are constantly shifting your focus.

When you are seeing the overall picture or getting a sense of a situation, you are engaged in broad-external concentration. Here you take in and assess information from the outside world. However, to analyze that data, you move into broad-internal concentration, where you are making sense of what you see and planning what to do next.

Your next move is to focus more sharply on the cues you need to perform your task, eliminating any distractions in your environment. This is narrow-external attention, where your task is mental rehearsal. The fourth type of concentration is narrow-internal. Here you turn inward again in order to act — your thoughts are directed to the action at hand and nothing else.

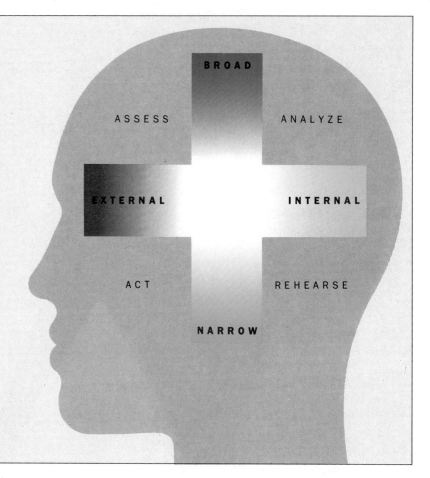

variable or environmental detail such as the weather or a road surface. Instead, they monitor and react to these conditions automatically as they occur.

Peak performance also seems effortless in that the athlete lets events happen instead of forcing them, and his or her actions are intuitive, automatic and unself-conscious. This release of conscious control over the mind and the body is the hallmark of the trained mind and skilled performers. Finally, for many athletes, a successful mental state is also linked closely to a sense of enjoyment, even exhilaration, that enhances their motivation and helps them to train hard over extended periods.

What gets in the way of reaching a peak performance?

In a survey of more than one thousand athletes of various ages and skill levels, the inability to cope with anxiety was the most frequent reason cited for failure to reach their potential. The anxiety reported by these athletes is divided into five categories: fear of failure; loss of control; feelings of inadequacy; guilt; and somatic complaints that are physiological indicators of anxiety such as sweating, muscle tension or an upset stomach. When any of these factors becomes excessive, it can manifest itself in both physical and psychological symptoms. These include a loss of coordination because of muscle tension, reduced flexibility, rapid heart rate, fatigue and a loss of concentration that results in being easily distracted, overly analytical and unable to stay interested in the activity.

Is a certain amount of anxiety necessary to get "psyched up" for a competitive event?
You need arousal, not anxiety, to sustain interest and concentration. Technically, *arousal* is a term that sports psychologists use to refer to the stress state, which can be thought of as the response a person undergoes whenever he or she encounters any change from the normal, balanced physiological state called homeostasis *(see illustration, page 9)*. As research into the causes and consequences of stress has repeatedly shown, people need some stress to function well. Studies of top athletes have indicated that prior to a performance they are not usually completely relaxed, but tend to exhibit various levels of physiological stress.

Some athletes require a high level of arousal to perform their best, while others do better when they are relaxed. The theoretical range of arousal levels that result in peak performances — perhaps unique for every individual — is called the zone of optimal functioning. First proposed by Soviet psychologist Yuri Hanin, this theory of optimal arousal is now widely accepted by American sports psychologists. If you fall short of this zone, you may be underaroused, a state that tends to be manifested as boredom, sluggishness and lack of interest. Or — as is often the case in competition — you may be overaroused, which is when anxiety becomes excessive. It is important to find your own optimal arousal level, which is different for each individual. Just what that level is depends not only on your personality but also on your skill level. Researchers have found that the more experienced a performer is, the greater his or her ability to handle physiological stress. In fact, skilled athletes need higher levels of stress to perform well, whereas beginners and moderately skilled athletes function best when calm and aroused minimally.

How do the techniques in this book help you attain optimal arousal?
One of the best ways to control overarousal is through the inward, meditative forms of relaxation described in Chapter Two. Meditation is not a passive state of rest like relaxing on a sofa, but a unique mental state characterized by reduced anxiety and heightened awareness. Meditation is cited by sports psychologists as a key element of mental-training programs.

Surprisingly, however, meditation can actually induce anxiety in some individuals. For them, other techniques such as progressive relaxation and the body scan, as described on page 25, can be effective substitutes for releasing stress.

While relaxation techniques can moderate overarousal before

One of the keys to staying with a sport or an exercise program — and enjoying it throughout your life — may be relinquishing the idea of winning and focusing instead on mastery. In a recent study of high school and college athletes, researchers found that young players whose only aim was winning tended to drop out of sports programs. Those who continued their activities were focusing on mastering their skills and improving their performance.

competition, many people find themselves underaroused during day-to-day training. This state can sap your motivation to continue with a workout or regimen, and it can cause you to perform lackadaisically in a competitive situation. Often you need to learn how to "psyche" yourself up. The section on motivation and goal setting on pages 20-21 shows how to use breathing techniques, positive feedback called self-talk, and reasonable short-term goals to increase your motivation level.

What effect does mental training have on the brain?

No one knows for sure, but the research is intriguing. One line of study focuses on the right brain/left brain connection. The brain's left hemisphere is the center of linear verbal, analytical and logical skills, while the right hemisphere is associated with spatial thinking, esthetic and visual tasks, as well as creativity and intuition. Studies show that you can impede your performance mentally when your left brain is dominant because the critical faculties can interfere and inhibit your overall concentration.

The theory behind training the mind is that the two sides of the brain can be taught to interact more harmoniously via certain physical and mental exercises. For example, scientists have found that guided relaxation, meditation and prayer states coordinate the electrical activity between the two sides of the brain, which may account for the sense of inner peace reported by people who meditate regularly. One eminent stress researcher — Dr. Herbert Benson of the Harvard Medical School — sees deep relaxation as crucial for balancing the left and right hemispheres of the brain, thus preventing the analytical left brain from increasing feelings of anxiety.

Does mental training reduce everyday stress?

Some psychotherapists prescribe "positive thinking" techniques in addition to aerobic exercise as antidotes to stress and depression. Physiologists have known for some time that vigorous exercise can reduce anxiety, depression and hostility, an effect that can last up to five hours after the workout is over. Now they are researching whether the effects of physical exercise on the brain can be increased or duplicated by certain kinds of mental exercise. Because brain activity is chemical as well as electrical, neurologists have been examining the role of the brain chemicals called neurotransmitters, the signals by which our brain cells, or neurons, communicate with one another and with the rest of the body. Approximately 60 of these substances have been identified, and many of them are directly linked to emotional states. The theory is that exercise increases the production of monoamines, a class of neurotransmitters which includes endorphins, norepinephrine, seratonin and dopamine. These substances have been shown to have an analgesic — or pain-killing — as well as a euphoric or calming effect. This may explain "runners' high," in addition to the calming effect that aerobic exercise produces. Scientists

Relaxation Response and Energy Use

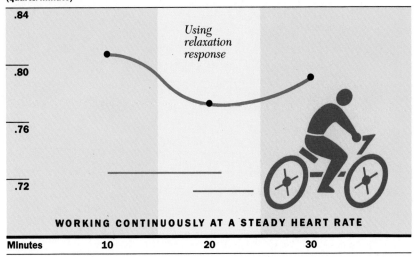

**Oxygen consumption
(quarts/minute)**

*Using
relaxation
response*

.84

.80

.76

.72

WORKING CONTINUOUSLY AT A STEADY HEART RATE

| Minutes | 10 | 20 | 30 |

To see if relaxation during exercise can lower energy expenditure, researchers in one study had subjects pedal a bicycle at a fixed rate for 30 minutes. During the middle 10-minute period the subjects used a meditation technique to relax, and their level of oxygen consumption — a measure of how hard they were exerting themselves — dropped 4 percent. The meditation, therefore, helped them perform the same amount of physical work with less effort.

are investigating the possibility that mental-training techniques might also trigger the release of certain monoamines.

Is mental training another phrase for self-confidence?

Since self-confidence must be based on the knowledge that you are well practiced in a skill, training your mind alone will not produce self-confidence. But it will help. Nurturing self-confidence and programming yourself with positive thoughts are practices that you can learn in a mental-training program. See pages 20-21 for information about how self-talk can help you change your self-image from unwittingly negative to positive.

A positive attitude seems to be an integral characteristic of winners. According to psychological profiles, top athletes tend to have a total belief in themselves and their abilities. Likewise, a study of high achievers in all fields shows that they have a very strong expectation of success.

Can you think your way to better performance?

One researcher linked runners to an electromyograph machine, which measures muscle movement, and had them imagine running up a steep hill. Even though the runners were lying still, the muscle groups involved in such a run were activated. Based on this study and a handful of other similar experiments, some researchers claim that the brain cannot distinguish between an imagined occurrence and an actual event. Therefore, thinking about a performance is mentally equal to doing it. Although this conclusion was widely reported in the press as reliable, as yet no study has substantiated it.

Even if they are not the equivalent of physical experience, visualization techniques — sometimes called imagery or imaging — have been effective in improving athletic performance. Visualization, or mentally rehearsing an event before you actually do it, is especially suited to sports or skills that allow time to plan ahead, or to anticipate and correct errors. For instance, an Alpine skier can benefit by taking the time to visualize himself making turns down his run while he is still at the starting gate. Although almost everyone visualizes future events to some extent, techniques to improve your ability to visualize effectively are given on page 18.

Does mental training involve hypnosis?

It can, but it need not. Hypnosis involves being put into an altered state of consciousness, a trance in which you remain mentally alert, somewhat like deep meditation. You will accept suggestions made by the hypnotist at this time — for example, that you are strong and accomplished enough to finish well in a race — more readily than you would accept them in your normal waking state. It can also affect how well you perform. In a study of weight lifters, for example, subjects were able to hoist a load 26 percent heavier than they were previously capable of lifting after being given the hypnotic suggestion that they could accomplish this.

However, hypnosis is not magic — you cannot achieve anything through hypnosis that you are incapable of physiologically. Some athletes use hypnosis to speed their progress in breaking through a mental barrier or sticking point, but the same ends can usually be achieved with other mental-training techniques and strong belief in your own skills and abilities.

Must you be an athlete to benefit from mental training?

No. Many people use mental-training techniques for self-improvement — to keep them on diets or give up smoking, or to prepare them for such challenges as giving a speech or presentation at work or just to foster self-confidence and feel better about themselves. Others believe that these practices can help them develop the discipline to begin or to stick with a fitness program. Using mental training, you can teach your mind to dismiss any negative thoughts that interfere with progress and substitute beliefs that will help you achieve your fitness goals.

How should you embark on a mental-training program?

Begin to train your mind by learning the techniques of relaxation described in Chapter Two. A program of Yoga can help you to use respiration and body position to enter a state of mental harmony as a basis for achieving optimal arousal. When you can control your arousal level, Chapter Three will explain how to develop your ability to focus entirely on your chosen activity. The Aikido exercises, which require intense focus, can help you increase your ability to enter into

Peak Performance: Imagery and Relaxation

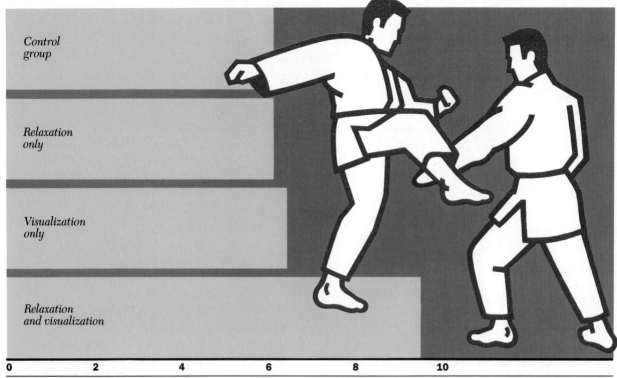

Control group

Relaxation only

Visualization only

Relaxation and visualization

| 0 | 2 | 4 | 6 | 8 | 10 |

Scores during competition

a flow state. The section on designing your own program beginning on page 16 will show you in detail how to use the techniques of goal setting, visualization, and self-talk.

How often should you practice mental training?

For best results, mental training should become an intrinsic part of your routine, which you practice regularly, like any other skill. There is no set rule as to how often or how long you should do your mental workouts. This will largely depend on which techniques you adopt and whether you choose to begin externally with such physical exercises as Yoga and Aikido; or internally with the visualization, goal-setting and positive-feedback techniques and guidelines described on pages 18-21.

Some experts advise practicing the purely mental skills at least three times a week. You may not see any results for two to three weeks, but as you continue practicing you will begin to notice subtle changes, including a feeling of being more attuned to your body. After making mental training a regular part of your life, you will be rewarded with the discovery of effective new ways of thought and behavior that will boost your self-esteem and improve the quality of your physical workouts.

Imagery, also called visualization, is the technique of imagining an event like a race or a game in as vivid detail as possible. That imagery works best to improve performance when combined with deep relaxation was shown by a study of Karate students. The class was divided into four groups: relaxation only, imagery only, a combination of these two disciplines, and a control group. When the students were given customary tests of skill in basic moves and sparring, the combination group scored noticeably higher than the others.

How to Design Your Own Program

The mental aspects of performance — avoiding unnecessary tension, maintaining concentration and staying motivated — revolve around being able to control your state of arousal, or stress. Arousal makes you alert and prepares you for action. But if your arousal level runs out of control, your performance can fall apart: you "choke" during an athletic event, go blank in the middle of an exam or stumble while giving a speech. When you try harder to cope with the anxiety, your arousal typically increases, which can make the situation even worse. The questions here will help you determine how well you cope with arousal, and suggest ways to improve your control of it.

How focused are you?

1 **Do you find it hard to focus unless you are competing?**

If you need the stimulation of competition to arouse yourself for exercise, you may find workout sessions boring or ineffective. In that case, you can get better results from exercise if you use the motivation techniques described in this book to help control your arousal level. Learning to motivate yourself and concentrate effectively can make a workout far more productive. For example, many champion body builders have noted that they attain superior muscle development when they have a specific mental image of the muscles they are exercising during a workout. Visualization, self-talk and the goal-setting tips described on pages 18-21 can all make your workouts more efficient as well as more interesting.

2 **When you compete, do you play to win?**

Competition is a stimulus to better performance — in sports and in life. It sharpens abilities and it can also be tremendously satisfying to experience. However, the athlete who thinks about nothing but winning is almost sure to lose. Overcompetitiveness breeds anxiety because too much is riding on the performance: If you make a mistake, if you lose, your self-worth is dealt a heavy blow. Anxiety interferes with your skills by spoiling your concentration. Successful athletes — and people who are successful in almost any field — enjoy what they do. They are not compelled to win to achieve fame and glory but compete for the fun of it. And they take satisfaction in practicing a skill as well as applying it against an opponent.

3 **Do you get injured often?**

If you train or compete regularly, then you have probably sustained at least a few injuries, particularly those caused by the cumulative stress of overworking muscles during exercise. Many people simply accept getting injured as a consequence of being physically active. But unless you engage in heavy-contact sports or train at intense levels, injuries that sideline you are probably avoidable. When regular exercisers get hurt, it is often because they fail to pay attention to their environment or to their bodies. Experienced athletes are attuned to the messages their bodies send them, and so are able to tread the line between improvement and injury. One of the best ways to build this type of centered awareness is through martial arts training, such as the Aikido routines shown in Chapter Three.

4 | Do you plan your strategy before a performance?

If you like to imagine yourself performing a task — whether you are playing a tennis match or delivering a speech — prior to actually doing the activity, then you already use mental imagery, a technique that most elite athletes use to enhance their performances. Some visualize themselves in action dozens of times to become more familiar with how their bodies feel during performance. Others imagine various scenarios that may take place so that they will be better prepared for any possibility. The key is to make the visualization as vivid and elaborate as possible. For other tips on how to visualize effectively, see page 18.

5 | Do you perform best when you are psyched up or calm?

The degree of arousal you need to perform at or near your potential is an individual matter. There are two guidelines that are helpful in assessing your own optimal arousal level. One is your skill level: the more skilled you are at an activity, the greater your tolerance for stress will be and the more arousal you may need to stay alert. Indeed, elite athletes are often highly aroused before an event — though their arousal is often manifested physically in gestures and rituals rather than in feelings of anxiety. The second guideline concerns how your arousal level should be tailored to the type of activity you are engaged in. Activities that rely on power, such as weight lifting or sprinting, utilize great arousal for peak performance, while activities involving fine motor skills — figure skating and archery, for example — are best performed in a relaxed state. Most sports require a combination of power and control, and to perform them well, you must adjust your mental skills as well as your physical ones. You will find tips on how to adjust your focus for specific activities in Chapter Four.

Visualization

In one survey of elite athletes, 98 percent reported that they employed visualization — the technique of imagining an activity before performing it. By focusing your mind, visualization — which is also known as imaging or mental rehearsal — helps to reduce anxiety and develop a state of relaxed alertness. Researchers now contend that when you visualize yourself performing, whether for a sport or a noncompetitive exercise, you are staging a dress rehearsal in which low-level sequences of electrical impulses are actually sent to your muscles, readying them for activity.

You can use imagery not only immediately before a performance, but also afterward as an instant replay, allowing you to re-experience a successful performance. Physiologists believe imagery can be a good way to establish the bodily association of how a peak performance feels. Many athletes also like to practice visualization just before they go to sleep. Some set aside time for mental rehearsal, and others engage in short visualizations whenever they have a few spare moments.

Not everyone visualizes in exactly the same way. Some athletes mentally watch a movie in which they are the principal actors; others visualize from the camera's point of view, so they "see" the environment and the activity but not themselves. Similarly, people's imagery can be so vivid it seems real, while others get less clear pictures or only sensations in their muscles. Any of these types of images can be effective; however, it is important that the visualization involves movement. Studies show that imagining still pictures will not help you perform better.

When you visualize, it is important to be relaxed: Relaxation increases the blood flow to the cerebral cortex, which is the center of visual imagery. Therefore, you should lie down or sit comfortably, loosen your clothing and close your eyes. Slowly and methodically relax all your muscles, starting with your face and progressing through your body to your legs and feet. Focus attention to your breathing, sensing your body as you inhale and exhale. Your body will gradually feel warmer and heavier. If your thoughts wander, bring your attention gently back to your breathing.

Once you are fully relaxed — it should take 10 minutes or so — picture yourself in whichever situation you wish to work on and patiently go through the step-by-step sequence of events. You should imagine every aspect of the game, including the sights, sounds and smells associated with your sport or exercise. You may experience your muscles mimicking the physical motions of your workout at a much lower intensity.

Try to rehearse the action or routine you are practicing just as you would actually perform it, with the same rhythm and tempo. If you want to imagine running a mile in six minutes, your visualization should last exactly that long. This is important, because you establish with imagery the same neurological patterns that will be required to do the activity. (There is one exception to this "real-time" rule: When you are learning a new skill or working on a particular problem, it can help to do your visualization in slow motion.)

Visualization Drills

To sharpen your ability to visualize, practice the following exercises, which have been developed by sports psychologists. (You will find examples of visualizations for sports on pages 110 and 118.)

• Begin by forming a mental image of someone or something. Exhale and relax. Examine what you are imagining in as much detail as possible. Concentrate on the image for about 20 seconds. Now erase the image from your mind completely by imagining a neutral space. After a few seconds, recall the original image. This may be difficult, but with practice it will become easier.

• Recall a moment in which you were successful in your sport, regardless of the ultimate outcome of the game. Choose a "trigger word," such as *slam*, to represent your memory and begin your visualization by saying the word to yourself. Keeping the time in your memory the same as that of the real event or slower, imagine the action in as vivid detail as possible. Allow your muscles to recall the feeling of your actions as you visualize them. When you have finished your visualization, repeat your trigger word.

• Visualize the performance of someone more skilled than yourself in a game or exercise situation. Be aware of the athlete's exact body position as he or she moves through the action. Then, in a practice session, act out the performance you have imagined.

Mind Over Muscle

This is an experiment that shows how your mind influences your muscles. Attach a key or some other light weight to a string and, with elbow bent and stabilized, dangle the device so that the key is directly above the center of the circle at right. Without moving your fingers or your arm, imagine the key making a clockwise revolution around the perimeter of the circle. Now visualize it moving counter-clockwise. You should see the key moving slightly in the pattern that you imagine. Next imagine the key moving like a pendulum along first one, and then the other axis of the central cross. Even with no real action occurring, your muscles are responding to the power of your mind to visualize the key's movement.

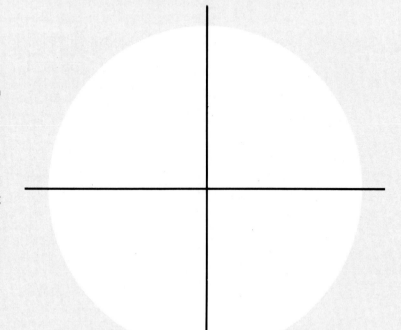

Staying Motivated

Most people begin a fitness regimen with the good intentions of losing weight, building strength and endurance, refining sports performance and improving health. However, many individuals find that good intentions are not enough to keep them on a regimen or off bad habits for long.

Fortunately, sports psychologists have developed a number of techniques to increase your motivation to continue exercise. These techniques are divided into two broad groups. The first category, known as cognitive methods, involves deliberate planning and conscious effort to think positively about exercise. The second group, behavioral approaches, involves structuring your environment so it is most conducive to staying with your plan.

Proper goal setting, a cognitive method, is one of the most important ways to motivate yourself. If your goals are unrealistic, or if they are too easy to attain, you can become bored with your program quickly and stop it. For tips on how to set goals that are most appropriate for you, see the next page.

Even though you may have a set of clearly defined and realistic goals, you may stop an exercise program because you perceive the costs of exercise are higher than the benefits. To determine your own costs-versus-benefits ratio, draw a line down the center of a piece of paper. On one side, list all the costs of exercise: time requirements, health club or equipment fees, self-conscious-ness about exercising in public. On the other side, list all the benefits: weight loss, improved cardiovascular endurance, increased muscle tone, stress reduction, better appearance, and so on. See if the costs can be reduced. For instance, you might find that exercising for 20 minutes a day, instead of a half hour three times a week only takes an hour and a half of your time per week — certainly a short time for improved fitness. If you think the health club fee is too high and you are self-conscious about exercising in public, consider buying a stationary bicycle for your home. Then you can reduce the costs of exercise and increase the chance that you will continue with a program.

Make it easy on yourself to exercise. You may find it convenient to combine exercise with other activities. For instance, if you live a few miles from your work place, perhaps you can walk or bicycle to your job, thus commuting and exercising at the same time.

If you feel tired or do not want to exercise on a particular day, start out with the intention of doing only half the duration or distance of your usual routine. Chances are, by the time you work up a sweat, you will decide to do a full workout after all.

Write a contract with yourself, stating your objectives. Then write down how you plan to achieve those goals. Sign the contract and give a copy to a friend or your spouse, someone who will encourage you if your resolve begins to erode.

Setting the Right Goals

Goal setting can be the key to staying motivated with an exercise schedule. Therefore, it is crucial that you set the right goals when you start a program. Also, if you have already begun a program but your enthusiasm is beginning to dwindle, the reason may be that your goals are unrealistic. The following goal-setting tips should help you revitalize your commitment.

SET ATTAINABLE GOALS.
Just as you should not make your goals so difficult that you cannot achieve them, do not set a goal that you can accomplish immediately. If your goals are too easy, you will soon become bored; if your goals are too difficult, you will get frustrated.

SET SPECIFIC GOALS.
Such generalized goals as, "I want to lose weight and get in shape," are too vague for you to know when you have reached them. Better goals may be to lose 15-20 pounds or to swim a mile.

IDENTIFY RELATED GOALS.
Do not write a long, haphazard list of goals. It is better to make a shorter list of goals that are related to one another. For example, if you want to get in better shape, your related goals may be to decrease your heart rate at rest from 75 to 65, to bring your blood pressure down to 135/90 and finally to reduce your body weight from 195 to 175 pounds.

EXPRESS GOALS POSITIVELY.
Goals phrased in a negative manner are known to have a dampening effect on attitude when you are striving for improvement. Goals such as "I hope I don't get beaten," or "I don't want to miss this shot" are less effective than goals stated positively, such as "I will play better than I did last week" or "I will finish the race." Positive goals not only promote the feeling that they are attainable, they also allow you to feel you can achieve success rather than avoid failure.

SUBDIVIDE LONG-TERM GOALS.
A series of attainable, short-term goals is not so intimidating. If you are a runner, you may decide to run a marathon (26-mile race) in order to stay motivated. To achieve this, you set a long-term goal of running 40 miles a week. A more immediate goal, therefore, would be to run 20 miles a week within three months and finish a six-mile race. An intermediate goal would be to run 30 miles a week in another three months and finish a 10-mile race. By chipping away in this fashion, a daunting goal that may take a year to achieve becomes manageable.

BE FLEXIBLE.
Do not give up or waste time criticizing yourself if you miss an exercise session. Make it up another time or substitute another activity. Also, if you see that you are going to fall short of a goal consistently, realize that goal was probably unrealistic in the first place and change it.

KEEP TRACK OF YOUR OBJECTIVES.
Record your achievements. Maintain an exercise diary so that you can match your goals against your actual daily performance. In this way you can chart your progress and ensure that you will set achievable goals and accomplish them.

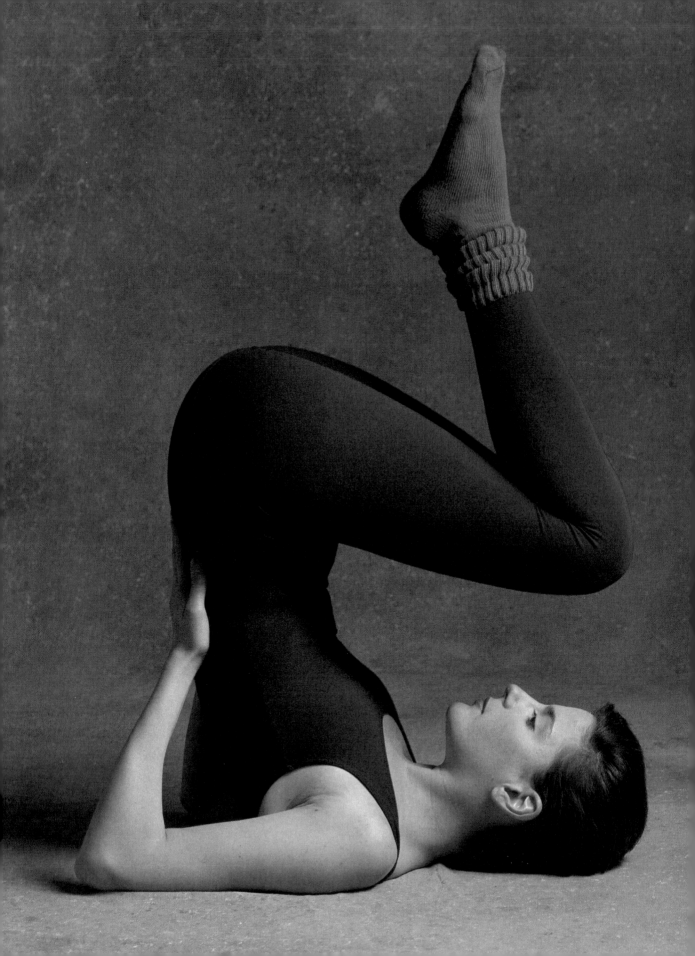

CHAPTER TWO

Relaxation

*Controlling arousal
with Yoga, deep breathing and
meditation*

Although most people think that relaxing is as simple as sitting down in front of the television, or lying on the sofa with your shoes off, in fact, relaxation is a skill. True relaxation is a state in which tension in your skeletal or voluntary muscles is reduced, and the activity of your involuntary muscles, which control such functions as breathing, heart rate and blood pressure, is also lowered. To achieve this state, you must first be aware of your body, since physical tension is linked inextricably to mental tension. Even such small actions as idly shaking your leg, pulling your hair or tapping your fingers are signs that you are not relaxed. Once you are aware of your tension, however, you will be able to use the relaxation techniques described in this chapter to reduce it.

For athletes, a common physical source of tension is the arousal that comes when they compete. To allow you to perform at peak levels, your sympathetic nervous system increases your arousal level by shifting your metabolism into high gear, making your muscles contract and your heart beat faster *(see illustration, page 9)*. But overarousal — too much muscle tension, a pounding heart, profuse sweating and butterflies in your stomach — will detract from your performance. You can control how aroused you become without sacrificing alertness by using the relaxation techniques of deep breathing, meditation and Hatha Yoga. Although the spiritual elements of these techniques have long been viewed with skepticism by pragmatic Westerners, the physiological responses they evoke are increasingly seen as valuable tools for controlling the sympathetic nervous system.

As Yoga and other Eastern forms of discipline and self-discovery like Zen meditation have gained wider acceptance by Western cultures, researchers have begun to subject them to scientific scrutiny. Their studies confirm that Yoga can help to relieve a variety of stress-related diseases, including hypertension, heart problems and ulcers. In light of these recent findings, the age-old claim that Yoga cures disease does not seem quite so farfetched as it once did.

The psychological effects of Yoga and meditation are more subjective and difficult to measure than the physiological, but several studies seem to confirm that Yoga helps reduce anxiety and resulting muscular tension. According to one three-year study conducted in India, the combination of meditation and Yoga can be useful for stress management. After six months of Yogic training, research subjects showed declines in nervous tension, respiratory problems, and drug and alcohol dependency, among other ailments. Other studies have shown that meditation can result in reduced oxygen consumption, lower serum cholesterol levels and a lower heart rate. Similarly, Zen practitioners have been shown to reduce their oxygen consumption by as much as 20 percent, which signals a substantial decrease in stress.

The physical fitness benefits of Yoga are among its most obvious and most easily proved. It is clear that assuming Yoga positions, called *asanas,* improves muscle flexibility and joint range of motion. Many athletic trainers and physical therapists have incorporated Yoga postures into fitness programs to enhance flexibility, reduce muscle tension and protect muscles and joints from injury. The Lotus position, for example, shown on page 28, stretches the inner thighs, the hips and, if you lean forward slightly, the lower back. Although many stretching exercises that condition specific muscles and muscle groups appear to be based on modern physiology, they are often derived from ancient Yoga asanas.

More passive forms of relaxation, such as watching television, daydreaming or taking a nap, cannot duplicate the benefits that Yoga and other forms of meditation can produce. Apparently, the meditative condition is a unique physiological state that is distinct from everyday diversions and other nonmeditative forms of relaxation. Electroencephalograms — tracings of electrical brain-wave patterns — have shown that when yogis are meditating, they may experience

Choosing a Relaxation Technique

In addition to meditation and Yoga, there are several relaxation techniques that have been shown to slow heartbeat and breathing and reduce tension and anxiety.

◆ *Progressive Relaxation.* You can practice this technique, which involves tensing and relaxing major muscle groups. Lie on your back on a mat with your arms at your sides and your palms up. Take a deep breath, hold it for a moment and then exhale, thinking of the word *relax*. Tighten your facial muscles as much as you can and hold for five seconds. Relax. Tighten the muscles in your shoulders, your arms and then your hands. Relax. Continue to tighten your muscles in groups and relax them, moving systematically down your body to your feet, ending with your toes. Finally, lie still, breathe slowly and imagine a peaceful scene.

◆ *The Relaxation Response.* This is a relaxed state induced by a simple meditation technique developed by Harvard Medical School professor Dr. Herbert Benson. Sit comfortably with your eyes closed and consciously relax all your muscles. Breathe through your nose, repeating the word *one* to yourself every time you exhale. Dismiss extraneous thoughts by thinking, "Oh, well." Continue to meditate in this way for twenty minutes. Remain seated with your eyes closed for several more minutes, then open your eyes for some additional minutes.

◆ *The Body Scan.* This technique combines breathing and focused awareness of muscle groups. With your eyes closed, inhale, mentally scanning your face and head for tension. As you exhale, imagine any noticeable tension draining away. Feel the tension decrease with every breath you exhale. Proceed to focus on your neck, shoulders, arms, stomach, chest, back, legs and, finally, your feet, scanning for tension when you inhale, and releasing the tension when you exhale. When you are finished, lie still for a few moments and be aware of your body's relaxed state.

not only reduced anxiety but also heightened awareness. Meditative techniques can be useful in situations where you want to relax effectively without any loss of concentration.

The exercises in this chapter are derived primarily from Hatha Yoga, the more widely practiced, physical form. Zen meditation can be practiced in any position, although many people prefer the Lotus or other such sitting positions as those on pages 28-29. These exercises can be done at any convenient time and as often as you wish, but many experts recommend doing them twice a day, once in the morning and again in the evening.

To practice Yoga and most other forms of meditation, you should find a quiet, comfortable place where you will not be interrupted. Remove jewelry and any clothing that is restrictive or binding. Sit on a carpet, meditation cushion or rolled exercise mat and remove your shoes. Do not practice meditation less than two hours after a meal, since the digestive process may disrupt your concentration and a full feeling may make you uncomfortable when you assume the Lotus or other Yoga positions.

Breathing

S low and controlled deep breathing is essential to relaxation. While rapid breathing raises the heart rate and elevates blood pressure, deep breathing is so powerful a relaxant that exhaling a single deep breath has been shown to reduce the heart rate.

During normal breathing, about 30 percent of the air you inhale stays in the nasal cavities and windpipe and 70 percent reaches the lungs. During deep breathing, however, 85 percent of the air inhaled is drawn into the lungs, allowing for a greater transfer of oxygen to the blood and expulsion of carbon dioxide.

Although most people take at least 17,000 breaths a day, they rarely think about the process involved. When you take a breath, the chest cavity expands outward as the ribs rise and, conversely, the diaphragm, a muscular partition between the chest and the abdomen, falls.

There are three basic types of breathing: diaphragmatic, the deepest kind of breathing in which your abdomen protrudes on inhalation; intercostal, in which the rib cage expands; and clavicular, the shallow breathing that occurs when you inhale air into only the top portion of the lungs. Breathing can involve all three elements. Performing the exercises on these two pages will help you become more aware of the three types of breathing.

Diaphragmatic breathing is the deepest form of respiration, yet most people avoid breathing this way because it requires relaxation of the abdominal muscles, causing the stomach to protrude. Lie on your back and relax. Exhale gradually but completely *(below)*. Inhale into the deepest portion of your lungs by allowing your stomach to extend out as you do so *(bottom)*. Exhale slowly and completely. Do not hold your breath.

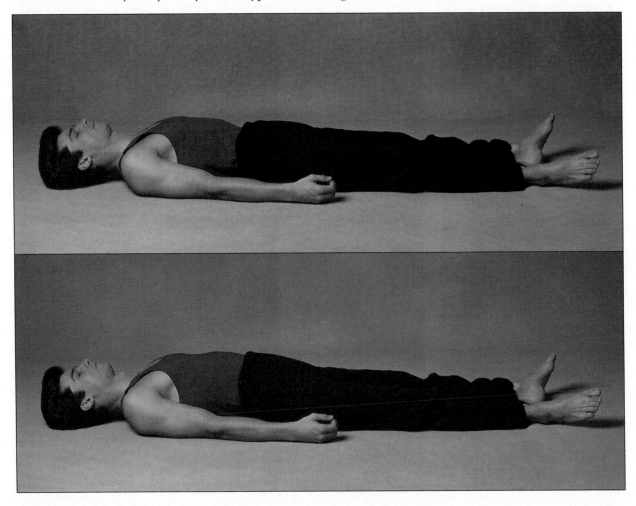

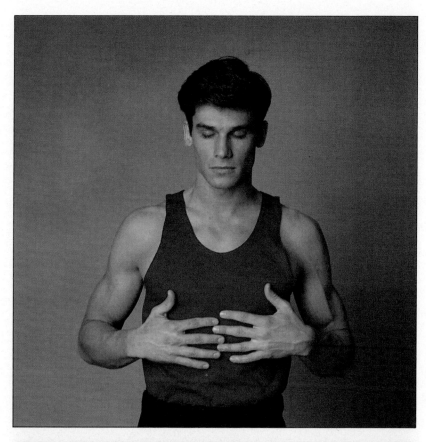

To get the feel of intercostal breathing, sit or stand up straight and exhale completely. Place the palms of your hands on both sides of your rib cage so that your fingers are interlaced slightly just below your breastbone *(left)*. Take a deep breath into the center of your lungs so that your fingers separate as if they were on the surface of an expanding balloon. Exhale.

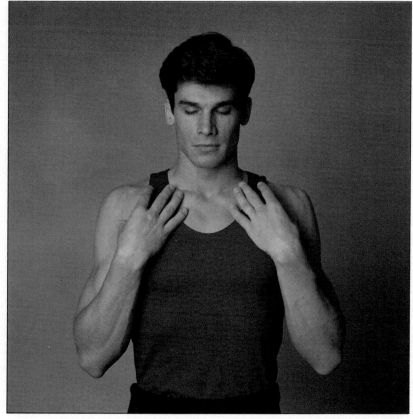

To become familiar with clavicular breathing, sit or stand with your back straight and place your fingertips just below your collarbone *(left)*. Inhale into the upper portion of your lungs so that your fingertips move up slightly toward your neck. This is the most shallow and least efficient breathing technique.

Meditation/1

The benefits of meditation are twofold: It clears the mind and relaxes the body. It has been shown to reduce muscle tension, heart rate, oxygen consumption and the metabolic rate. Meditation can be a useful relaxation tool as part of your preparation for physical or mental effort. It can also help you unwind afterward. However, you should not meditate just before or after a period of intense physical activity.

To get the most benefits from a meditation session, find a quiet place where you will not be distracted. Use any of the postures or hand positions shown on these two pages or the following two. Keep your eyes open, focusing on a spot three to four feet forward and downward. Use diaphragmatic breathing, as explained on page 26.

Think of a few words or sounds, such as the Yoga *om,* that have a calming effect on you and repeat them in a rhythmical cadence with your breathing. Focus only on those words and the depth of your breathing for approximately 15 minutes.

It takes time to learn proper meditation technique, so do not be discouraged if your mind wanders at first. With experience, you will find your concentration improving.

When you are ready to resume your usual activities, slowly move out of the meditative posture. If you cross your left leg over your right in your meditation session, cross your right leg over your left the next time.

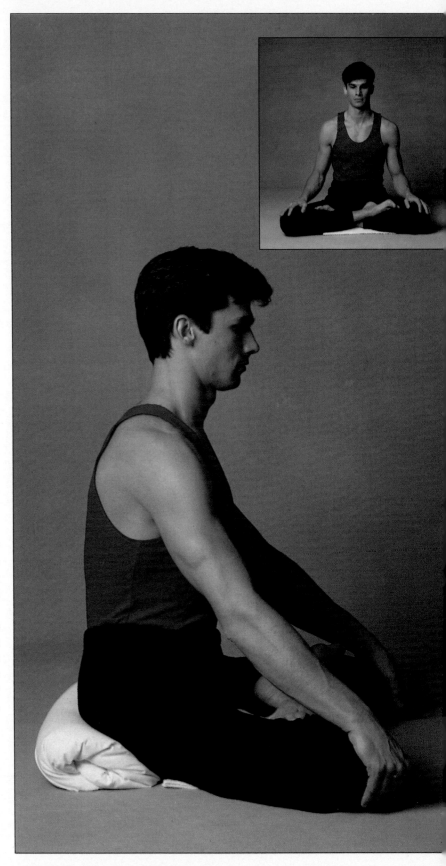

To meditate in the classic Lotus position, sit cross-legged on the floor. Wedge a pillow beneath you so that your pelvis is tilted forward slightly and your back is straight *(right),* with each foot placed on the opposite thigh and your hands on your knees *(inset).*

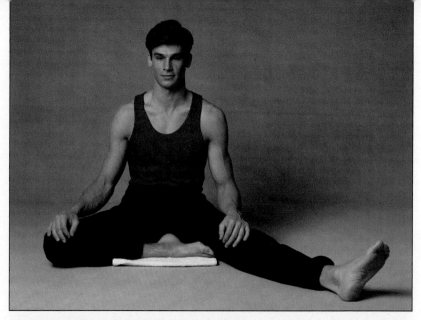

For an easier variation of the Lotus, sit with a pillow beneath you as you would in the Lotus position. Extend one leg and draw the other foot up to reach the inner thigh of the extended leg. For comfort's sake, place a towel under the foot that is closest to you.

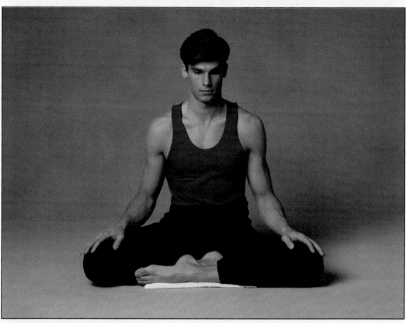

Another Lotus variation is the seated double-leg fold. Sit on the floor with a pillow beneath you and cross your legs as shown. Place a towel under your feet so you are comfortable and rest your hands on your knees.

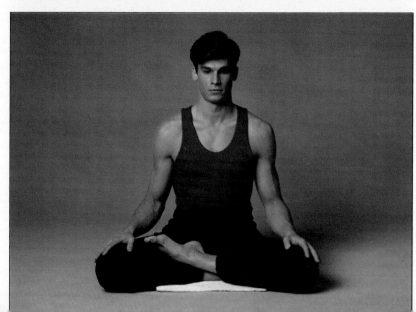

The half-Lotus is a meditative position preferred by people who find the full Lotus difficult to do. Sit cross-legged with a pillow beneath you. Place one foot on the opposite thigh and let the other foot rest on a towel.

Meditation/2

To use the traditional Hatha Yoga hand position, for the Lotus or any variation, place the backs of your hands on your knees, palms facing upward. Keep your fingers relaxed and touch the tips of your thumbs and index fingers *(right)*.

Cup your hands, press your thumbs together and place the outside edges of your hands on your abdomen for a Zen meditative position *(opposite)*.

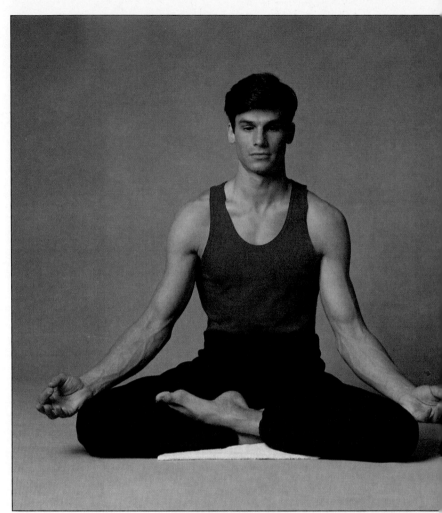

For a Tibetan meditative position, place the backs of your hands comfortably on your knees and position your thumbs on the first joints of your ring fingers *(right)*. Bend your fingers over your thumbs *(center)* and rotate your hands so that your palms face downward *(far right)*.

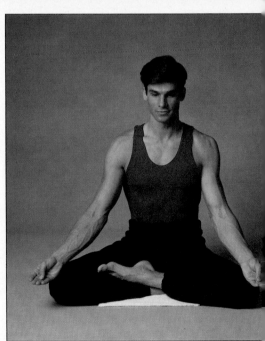

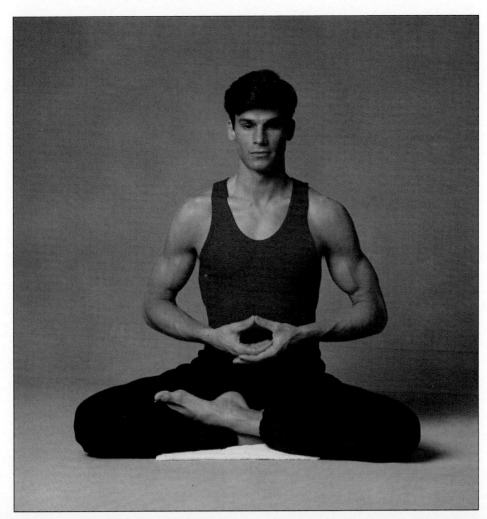

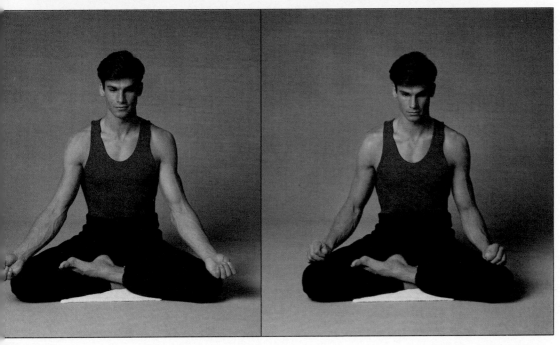

Warm-Ups/1

Yoga is an active exercise that requires some degree of flexibility and considerable joint range of motion. Trying to assume a difficult asana, or Yoga posture, is all the more taxing if you have not warmed up properly. The greater your flexibility, the easier it will be to achieve the Yoga asanas. Even if you are fairly flexible, you will often experience daily fluctuations of the limits of your range of motion. No matter how flexible you are generally, you should perform some warm-up exercises to loosen up prior to Yoga sessions.

The exercises on these two pages and the following two will contribute to enhanced flexibility, particularly in the hips, trunk, shoulders and spine. The exercises have been arranged in order of increasing difficulty, and they stretch complementary muscle groups. Take five to 10 minutes to do them before your Yoga sessions. Perform each warm-up on both sides of your body to ensure increased mobility.

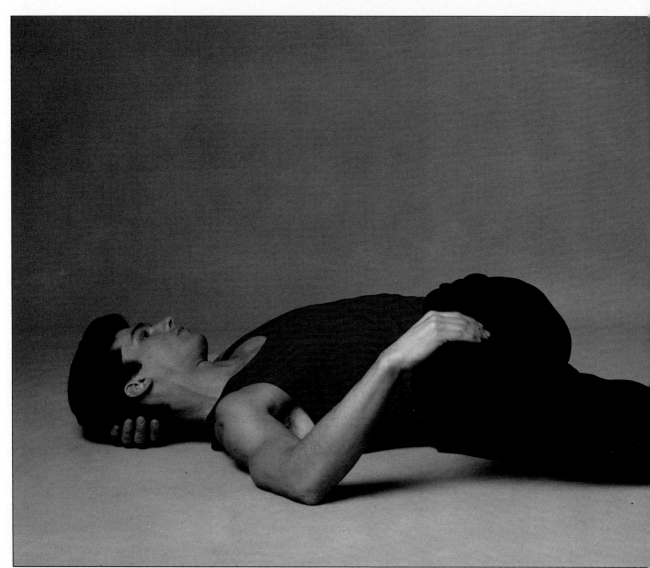

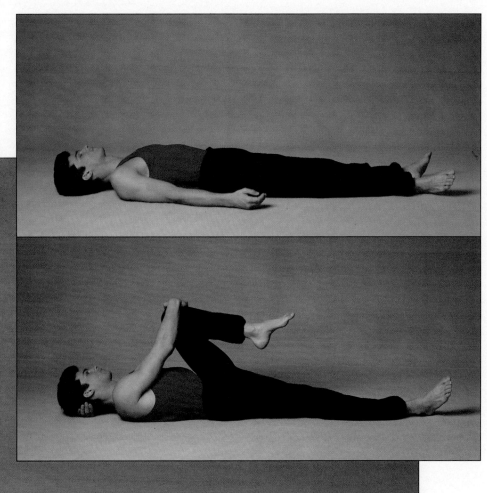

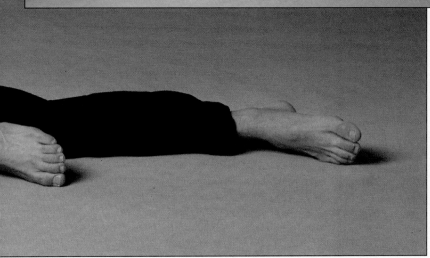

Lie on your back with your arms at your sides *(inset, top)*. Breathe diaphragmatically to relax, as shown on page 26. Then place your left hand under your head and draw your left knee toward your chest with your right hand *(inset, bottom)*. Keep both shoulders and left elbow on the floor and your right leg extended. Cross your left knee to the right side and pull it toward the floor *(left)*. You will feel a stretch along the back of your upper leg, hip and lower back, but it should not be painful. Repeat the movement for the right leg.

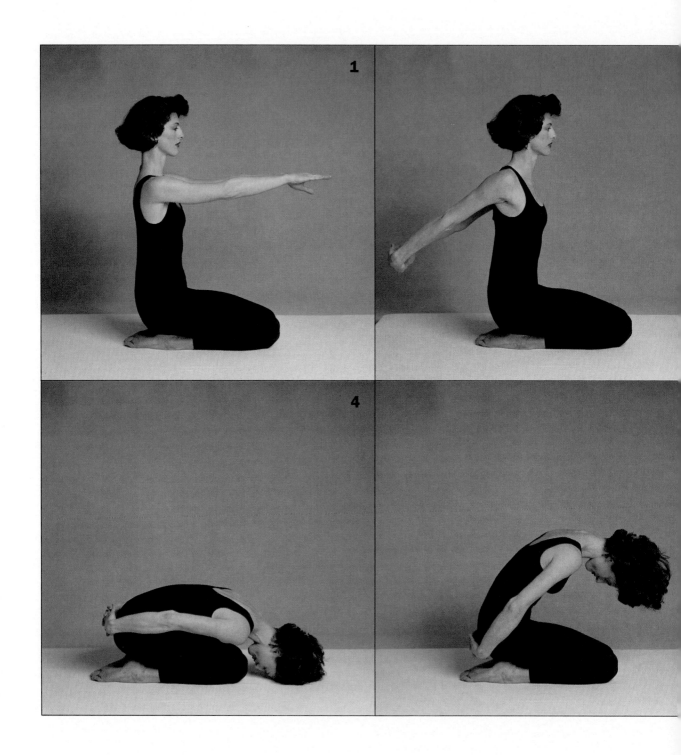

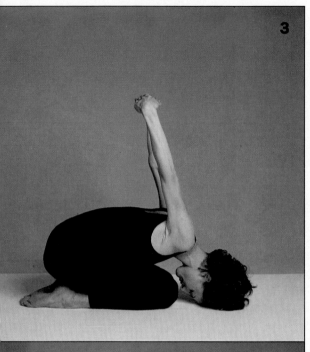

Warm-Ups/2

Kneel on the floor and sit on your heels. Keep your back straight and extend your arms and hands in front of you (1). Extend and rotate your arms behind you and interlace your fingers (2). Bend over so that your forehead touches the floor and your arms reach toward the ceiling (3). Bring your arms down and rest your hands on your buttocks (4), then gradually lengthen your torso upward, beginning from your lower back (5) until you are sitting erect again. Rest your hands at your sides (6).

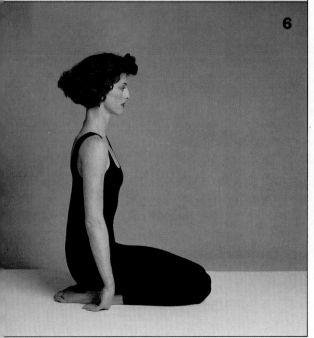

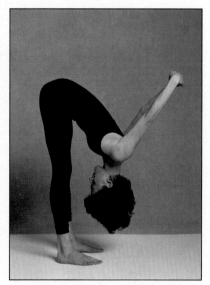

To perform the same mobility exercise from a standing position, follow the six steps in the same manner, making minor adjustments. The photograph above corresponds to step 3.

Yoga Asanas

Many practitioners of Yoga believe that an asana purifies the mind and body through a series of steps. The first of these is the strengthening of the body as you condition your muscles to assume a particular posture. When you have perfected the asana, your body adjusts to the posture and becomes steady; breath control and concentration contribute to your tranquility and a sense of physical comfort. Finally, through meditation, tranquility leads to heightened perception and self-awareness.

Do not rush through your asanas: Perform them slowly and smoothly. Do not daydream but think about your posture and visualize your body position. Breathe normally as you assume a posture and exhale as you bend forward or move deeper into the posture. If you perform a Yoga asana that stretches and strengthens the muscles of one side of your body, repeat the posture so that you stretch the other side as well.

The names of many of the Yoga positions shown in this chapter are English translations of the original Sanskrit words.

DOWNWARD-FACING DOG Kneel on an exercise mat with your feet hip-width apart and your hands spread about shoulder-width. Extend your buttocks toward the ceiling *(inset)* and straighten your legs. Do not lock your knees. Your back, arms and head should form a straight line. Lift one leg at a time so that you extend that line *(right).*

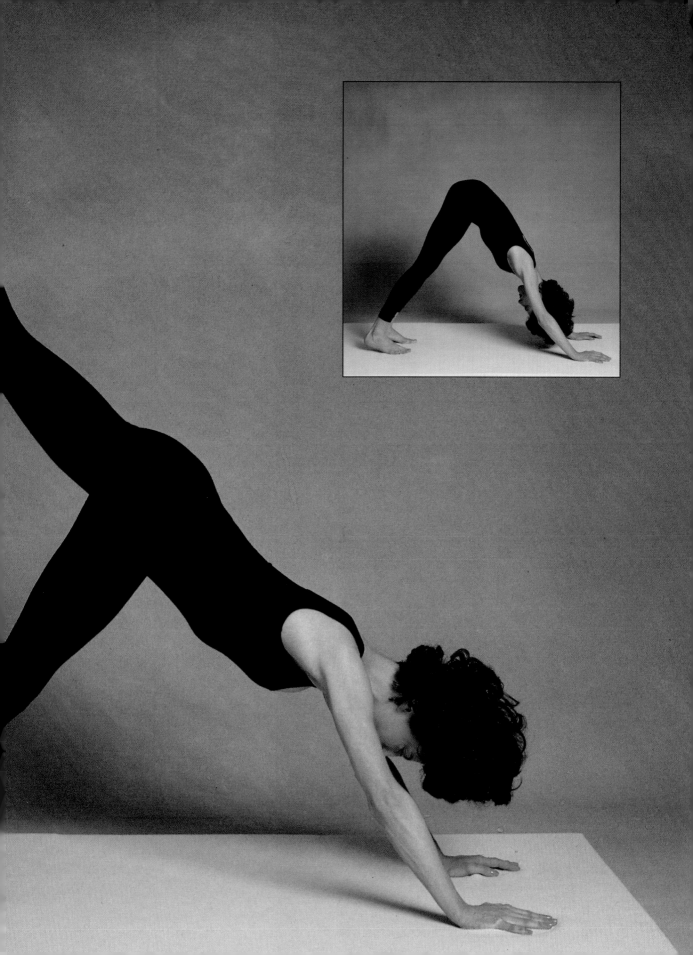

Sun Salutation

Stand erect with your feet about 12 inches apart and your hands at your sides. Do not lock your knees (1). Bring your palms together in front of your chest (2), and rotate your forearms and hands outward slowly so that the backs come together (3). Circle your hands inward until the fingers point downward (4). Continue the rotation and extend your elbows so that your palms face toward your feet (5). Circle your arms while reaching your hands back toward the ceiling, expand your chest and look up as if greeting the sun (6).

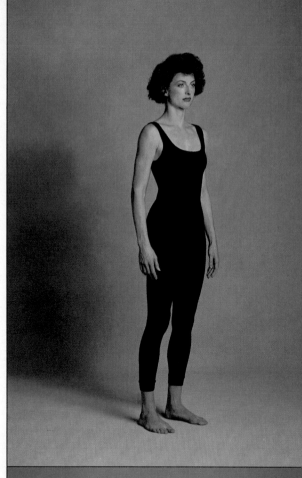

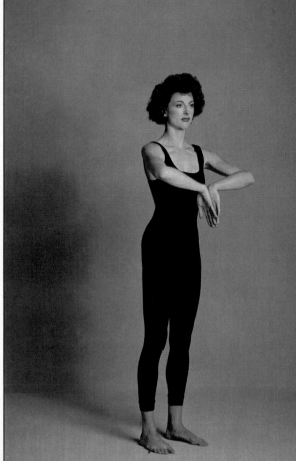

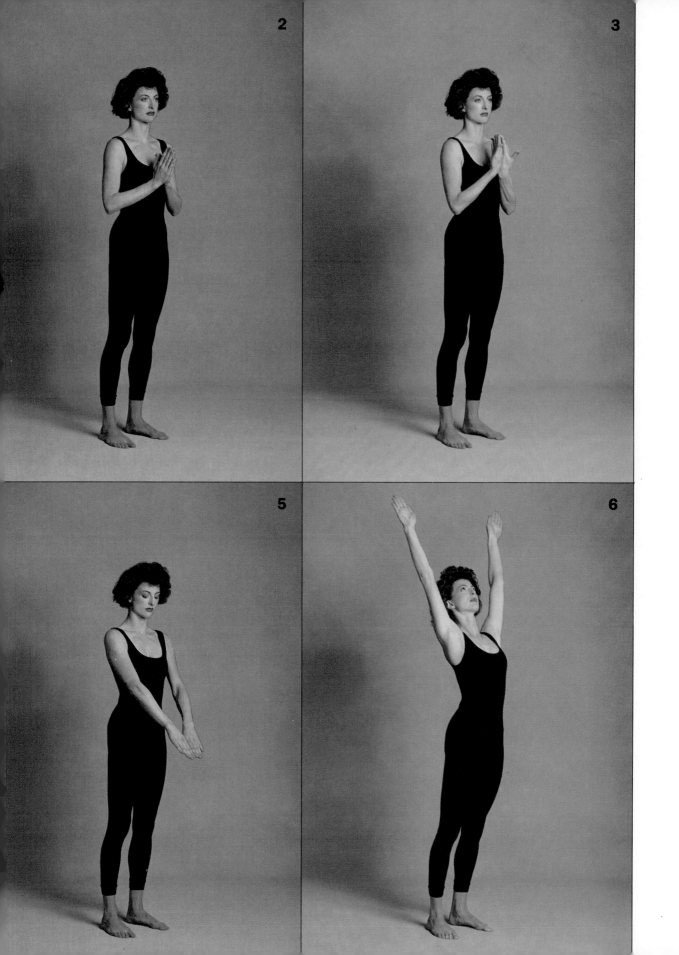

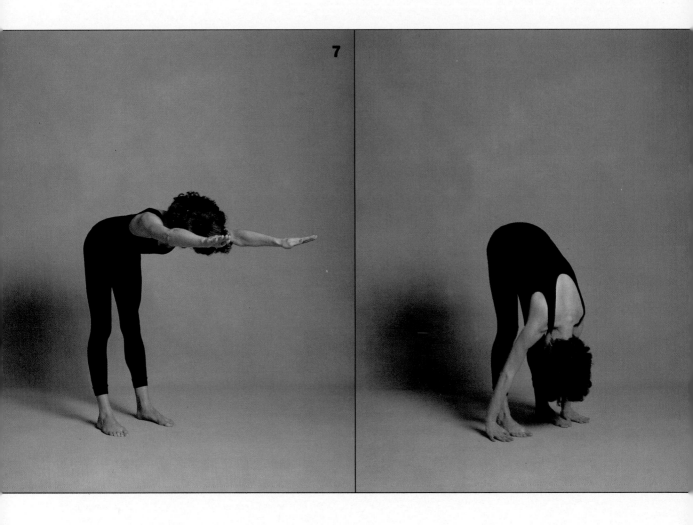

7

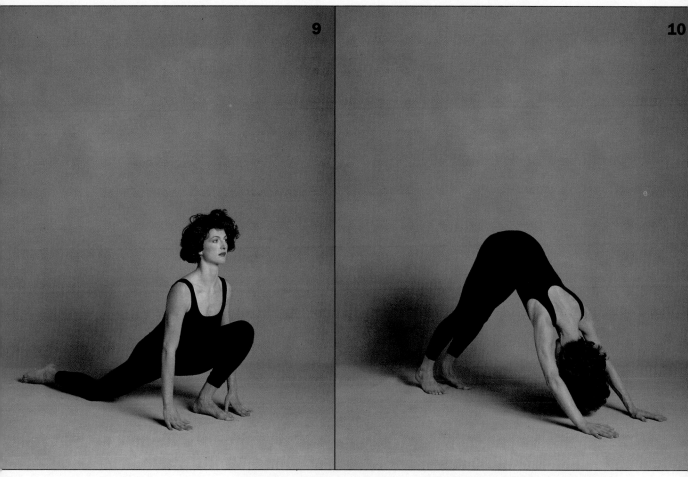

Bend forward at the hips with your arms extended to form the Table, in which your arms, back and head are parallel to the ground (7). Continue the downward movement. Keep your knees as straight as possible without locking them; place your palms on the floor next to your feet so that you are in the standing Folded Leaf posture (8). Bend your left knee, extend your right leg, expand your chest and assume the Horse and Rider position (9). Move into the Downward-Facing Dog by extending your left leg and lifting your buttocks toward the ceiling (10).

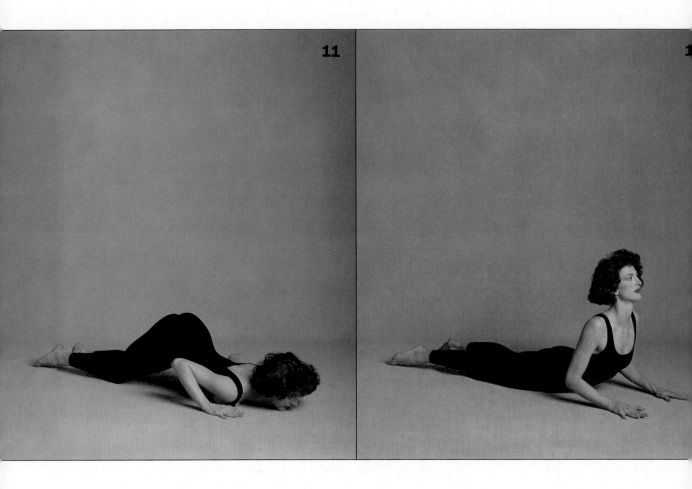

11

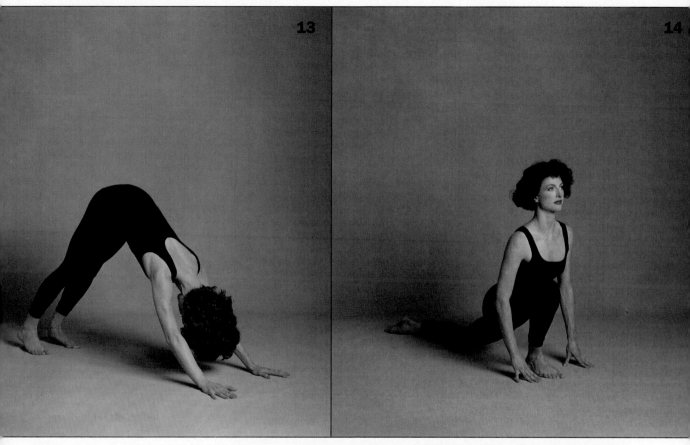

Keeping your buttocks raised, shift your weight toward your hands. Lower your knees and chest to the floor so that you are in the Cat position (11). Lower your thighs and hips so that they make contact with the floor and raise your chest into the Cobra (12). Reverse the procedure and return to the Downward-Facing Dog (13) and Horse and Rider, drawing your right leg forward, then extending your left leg (14).

SUN SALUTATION *(continued)*

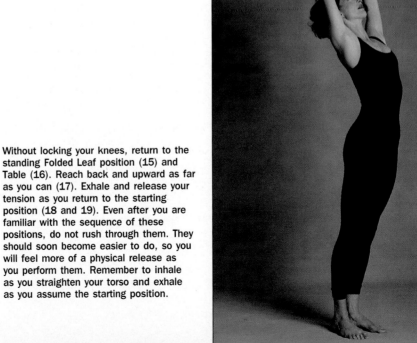

Without locking your knees, return to the standing Folded Leaf position (15) and Table (16). Reach back and upward as far as you can (17). Exhale and release your tension as you return to the starting position (18 and 19). Even after you are familiar with the sequence of these positions, do not rush through them. They should soon become easier to do, so you will feel more of a physical release as you perform them. Remember to inhale as you straighten your torso and exhale as you assume the starting position.

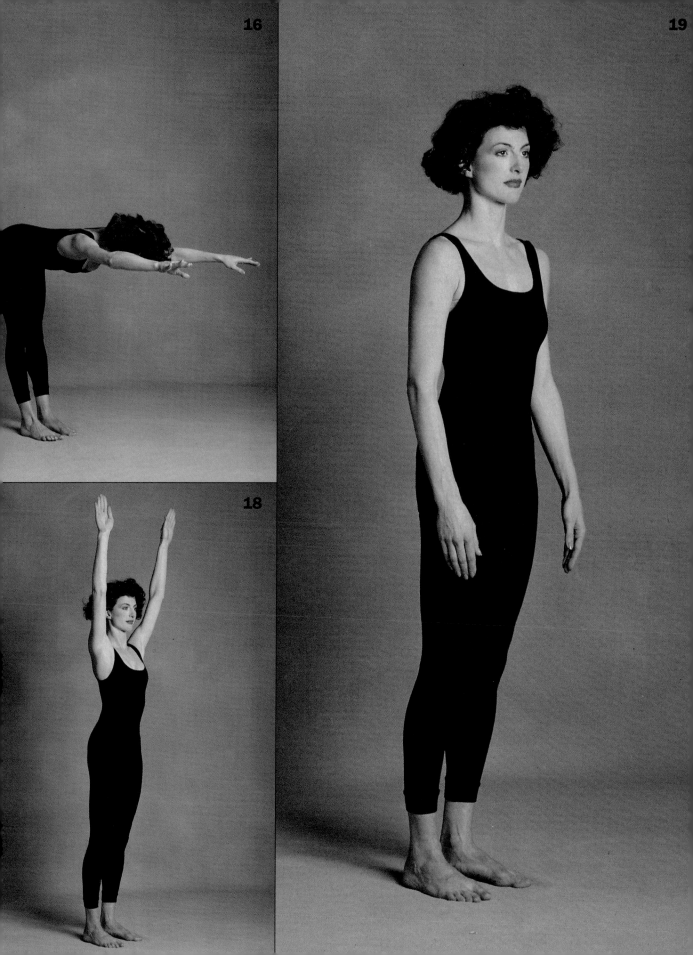

16

18

19

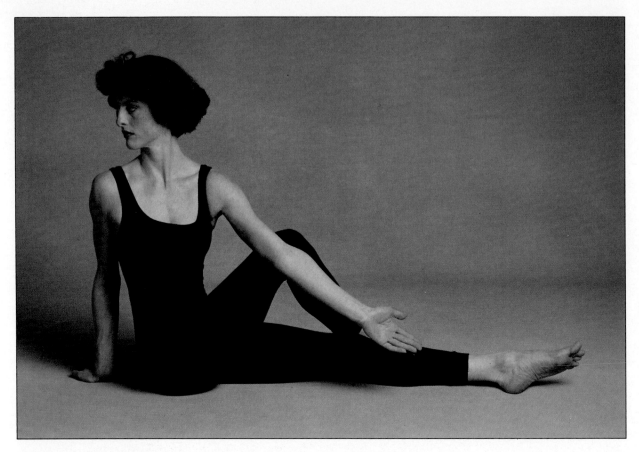

Spinal Twist

Sit on the floor, extend your left leg and cross your right leg over it above the knee. Supporting your upper body with your right arm, place your left elbow against your right knee. Fix your visual focus as far right as possible.

For a more advanced Spinal Twist, bend your left knee so that your heel touches your right buttocks and place your right hand behind your back *(inset)*. Hook your left arm under your right knee and clasp your fingers or hands behind you if possible. A small towel may be grasped instead *(right)*.

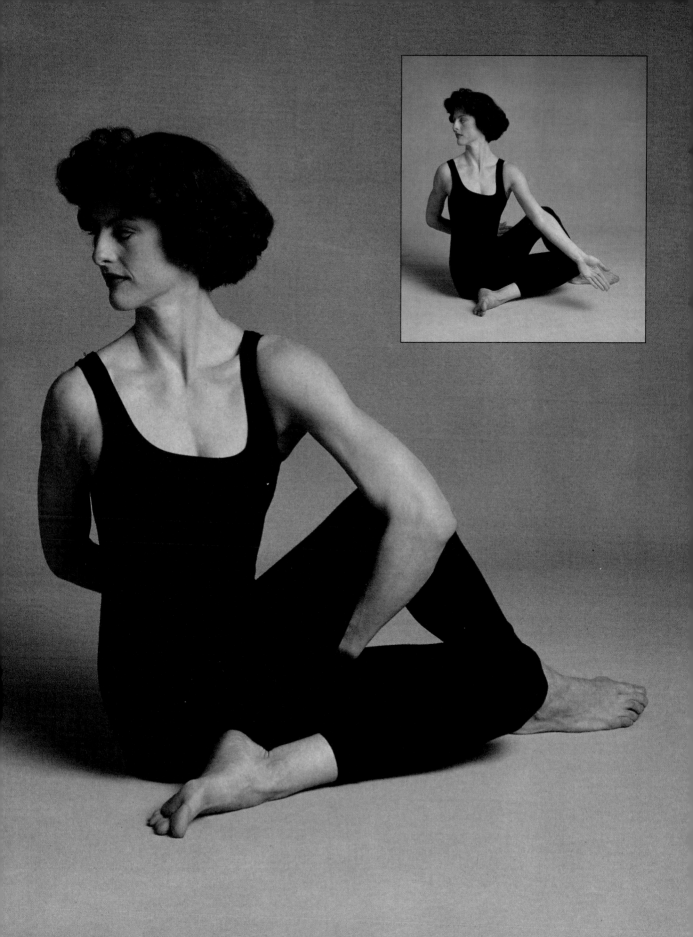

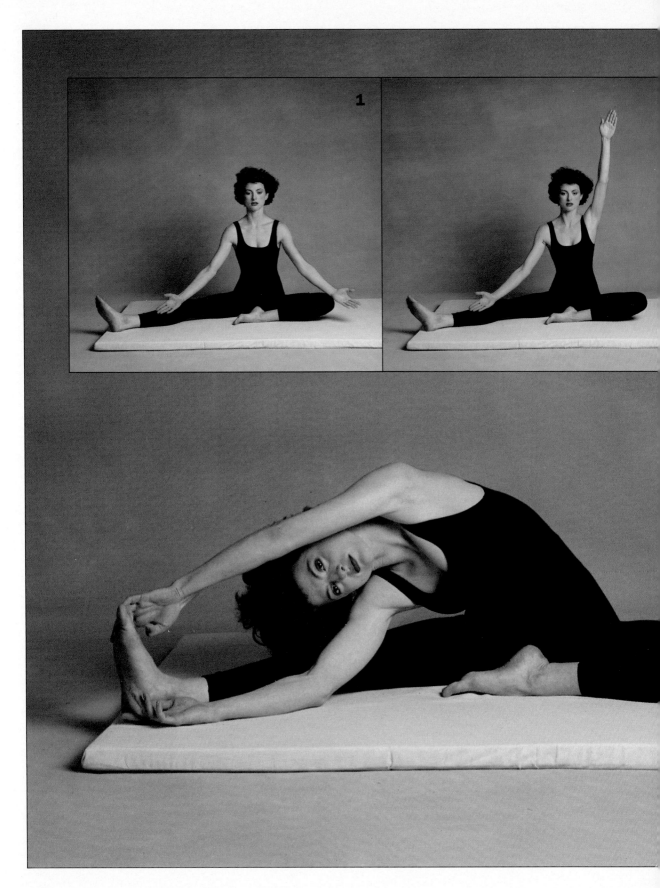

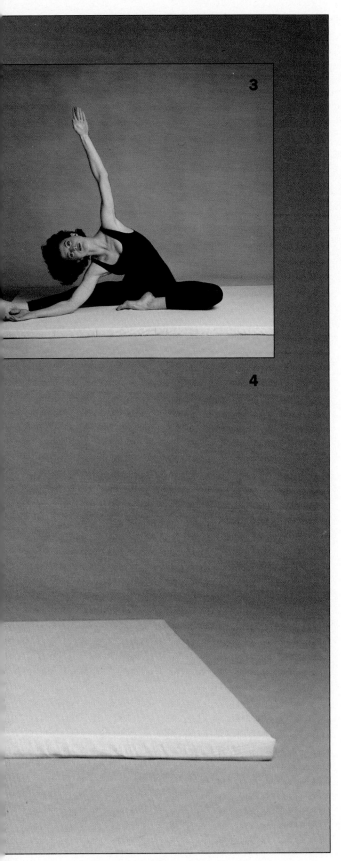

Head to Knee

Sit on the floor with your right leg
extended and your left heel drawn inward
to your right thigh and in line with the
center of your body. Extend your arms
wide with your palms up (1). Raise your
left arm and hand toward the ceiling (2).
Keeping your left hand up, slide your
right hand toward your right foot as you
extend your torso over your right leg (3).
Arc your left hand and arm toward your
right foot, exhale and lower your right ear
toward your right knee (4). To return to
your original position, reach your left arm
upward to the ceiling, gradually moving
up from your hips, through your rib cage,
then head until they line up vertically.
Bring your left hand downward until you
have assumed the original position.

Dove

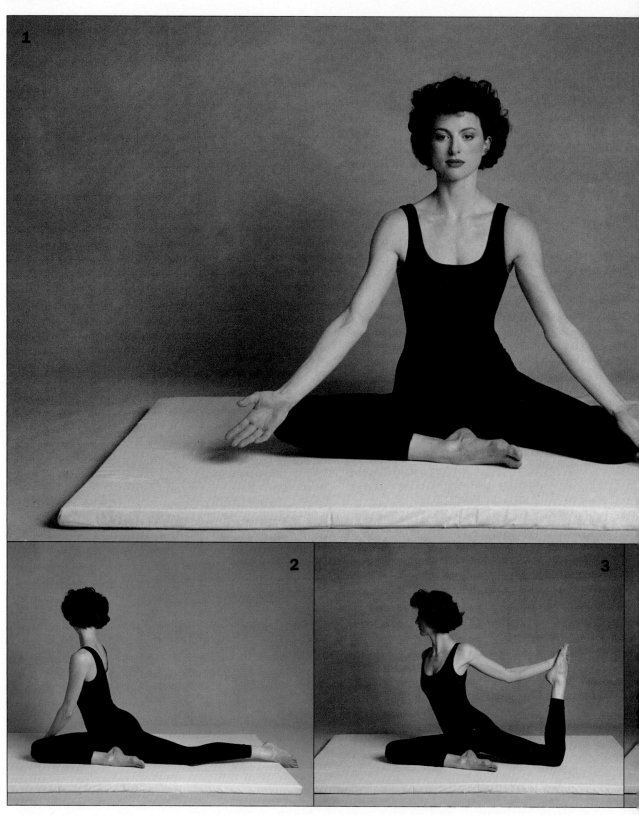

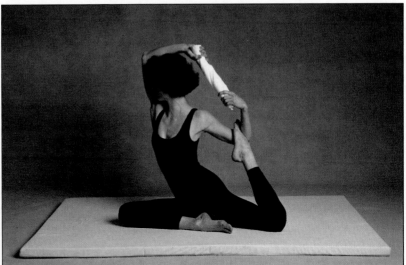

As a variation on the final Dove posture at left, hold a towel between your hands to help you maintain a steady position, as well as to increase your overall degree of stretch and flexibility.

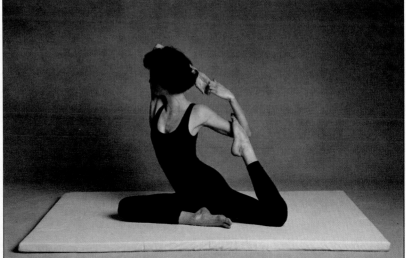

For a more advanced variation on the Dove position at left, interlace or hook your fingers and hold your hands or fingers together for additional stretch.

Sit on the floor with your right leg bent and drawn toward your left thigh with your right heel at the center line of your body. Bend your left leg behind you. Keep your back erect and widen your arms into an open position (1). Rotate to the right, extending your left leg and placing your hands on the floor to the outside of your right knee (2). Flex your left leg behind you and grasp your foot with your left hand (3). Draw your left heel toward you and bend your right elbow, pointing it toward the ceiling (4).

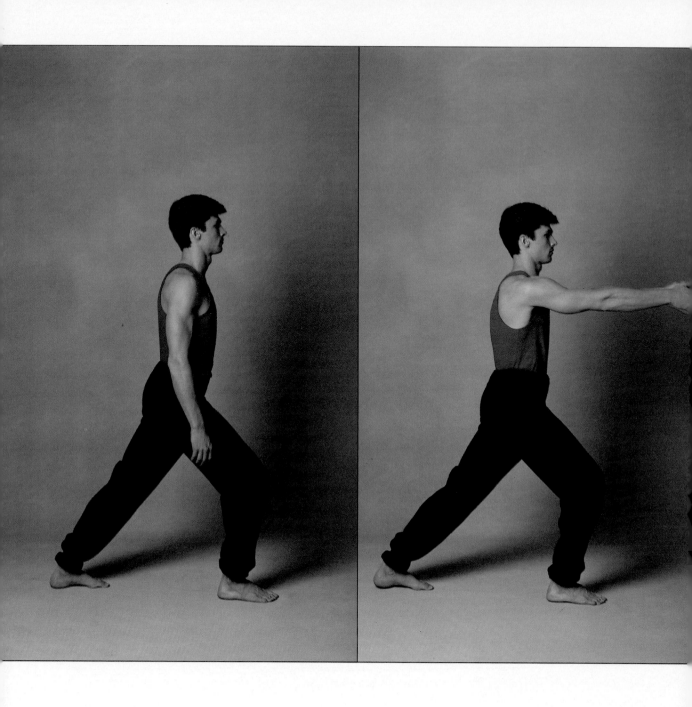

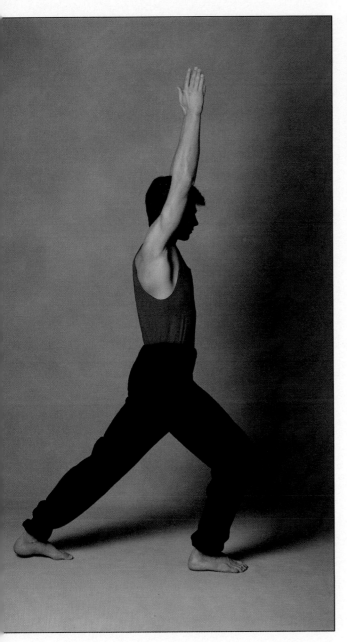

Warrior

Stand erect with your arms at your sides and and shift your weight forward, stepping your right foot into a lunge position *(far left)*. Keep your head and torso as vertically erect as possible. Extend your arms directly in front of you, shoulder-width apart, with your palms facing each other *(center)*. Lift your hands toward the ceiling, increasing the depth of your lunge and breathing *(left)*.

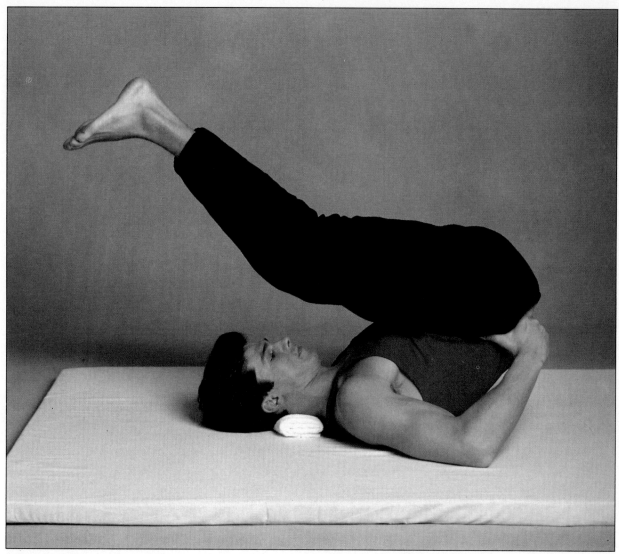

Shoulder Stand

For a half-shoulder stand, lie on your back with a towel folded under your neck for comfort and support. Lift your hips with your hands, supporting your body weight on your shoulders and upper arms. Extend your legs so that your knees are directly over your head *(above)*.

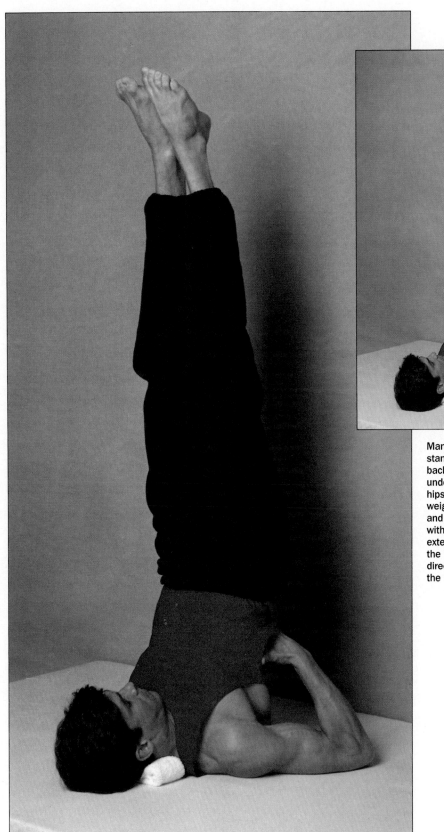

Many people find a complete shoulder stand difficult to do at first. Lie on your back very close to a wall. Place a towel under your neck for comfort. Support your hips with your hands so that your body weight is distributed on your shoulders and upper arms. Slowly walk up the wall with your feet (inset). When your legs are extended, carefully pull them away from the wall so that they are suspended directly over your body and point toward the ceiling (left).

Fish

Lie on your back with your arms at your sides *(inset)*. Pull your shoulder blades inward toward your spine and draw your elbows toward your sides, then roll your head far back enough for your shoulders to lift off the floor *(below)*. Be sure to keep your hips on the floor.

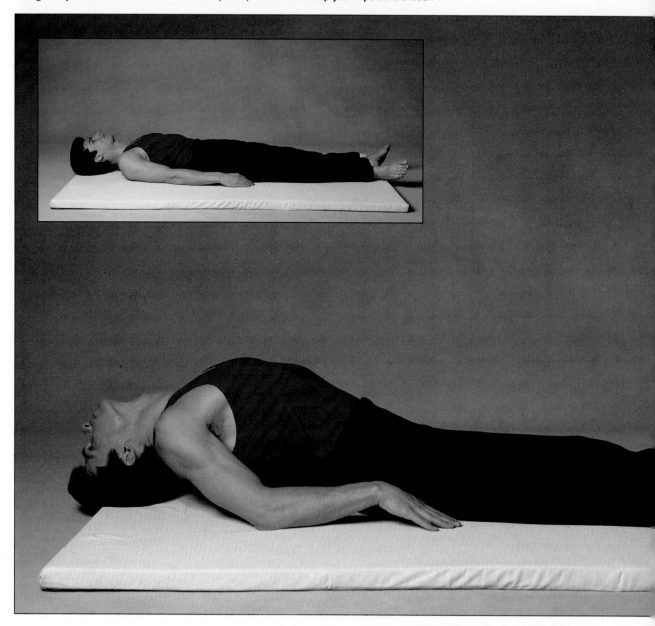

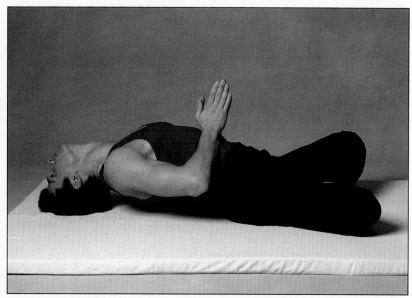

For a more advanced version of the Fish at left, lie on your back and place your legs into a half or full Lotus position. Support your upper body with your elbows and the top of your head *(left).*Then, supporting your upper torso with your head and your lower torso with your pelvis, lift your elbows off the floor and place your palms together over your abdomen *(above).*

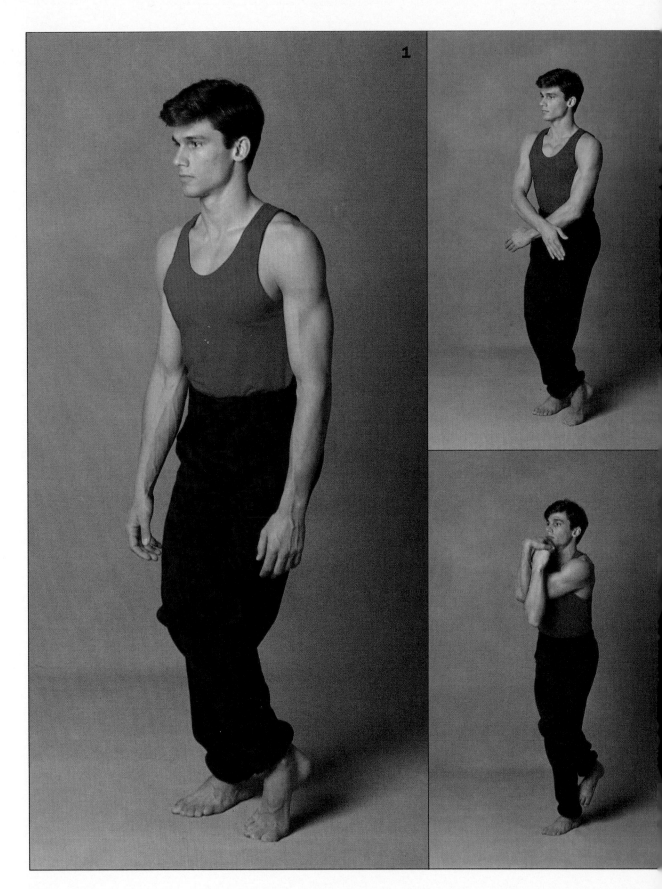

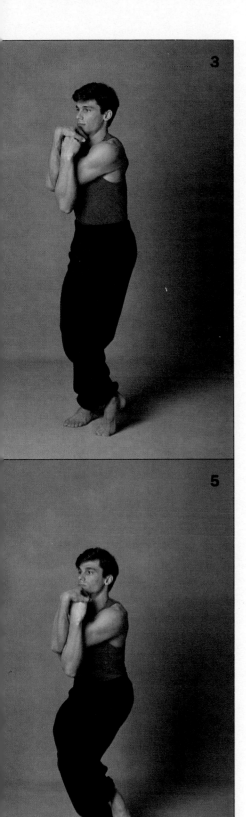

Eagle

Stand erect and cross your right foot in front of and to the left of your left foot (1). Cross your arms in front of you (2), then bend your left elbow around your right arm, with the back of your left hand into your right palm as shown. Bring your hands together under your chin (3). Lift your right foot off the floor and balance yourself on your left foot (4). Keeping your right leg crossed over your left, bend your left knee as much as you can with your pelvis over your left foot to help maintain your balance (5). Focus your gaze on a point three to four feet in front of you for greater stability.

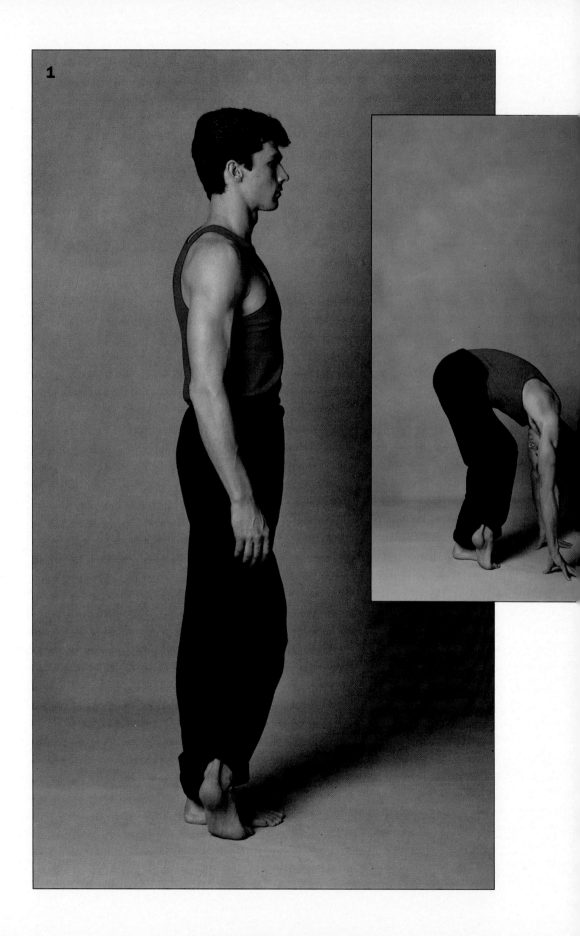

1

60

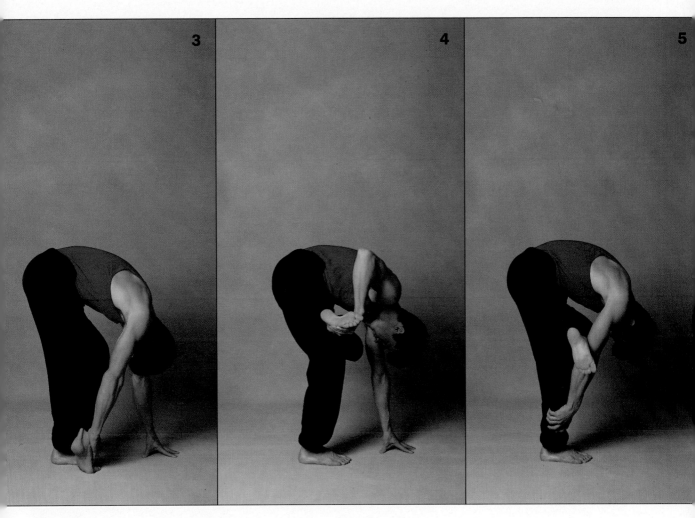

Stork

Stand erect and cross your left foot in front of your right. Place the toes of your left foot on the floor, pointing them toward your right foot (1). Bend over at the waist and hips and place your hands on the floor to steady yourself. Bend your right leg (2). Grasp your left foot with your right hand (3) and pull it upward and support it on your right knee or thigh (4). Release your left foot carefully and take your other hand off the floor. Grasp your right ankle with both hands (5). To return to a standing position, lower your left leg and uncurl slowly and smoothly to avoid feeling dizzy.

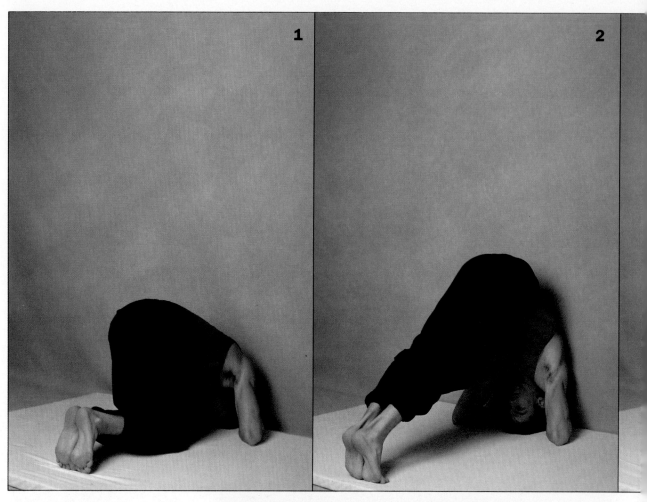

Headstand

Do not attempt this position if you have high blood pressure or a cardiac condition. Kneel on a mat in front of a wall, interlacing your fingers behind your head and supporting the weight of your upper body with your head and forearms (1). Extend your legs so that your upper body touches the wall and your lower body is supported by your extended legs and toes (2). Reach your right leg and foot back upward until it touches the wall (3). Then bring the left foot up and walk up the wall until both legs are extended. Carefully draw your legs and feet away so that your body is self-supporting on your arms and the top of your head (4).

To descend safely from the headstand, bring your feet back to the wall. Drop one leg down *(right)*, then the other. Curl into a resting position with your knees under your body and your arms at your sides *(far right)*. Remain in this position for a few minutes, and then rise slowly to avoid dizziness.

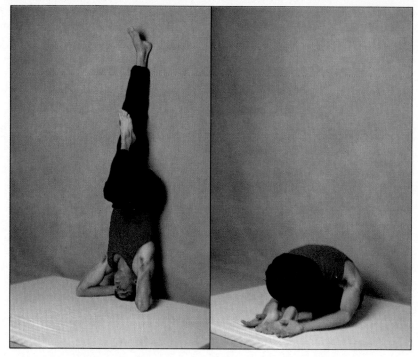

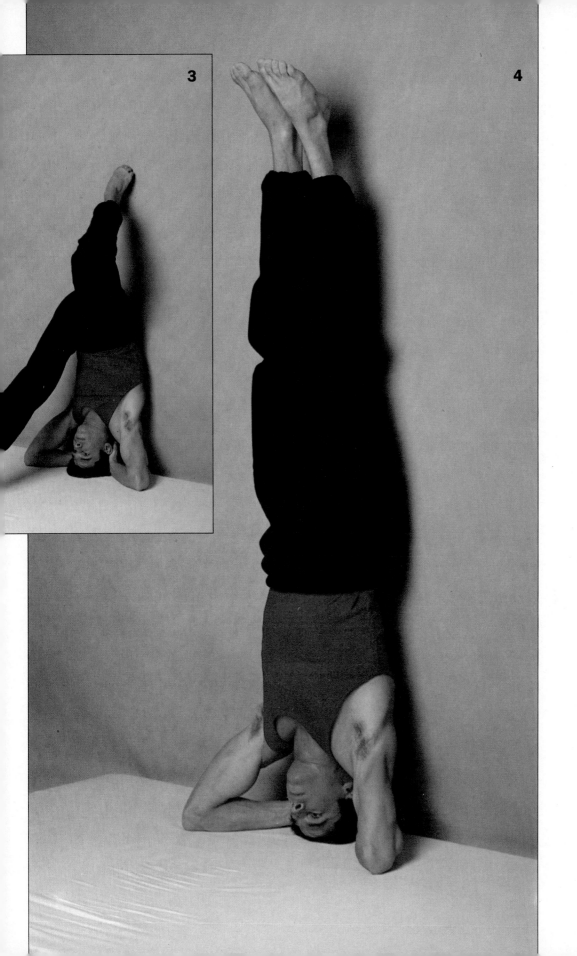

3

4

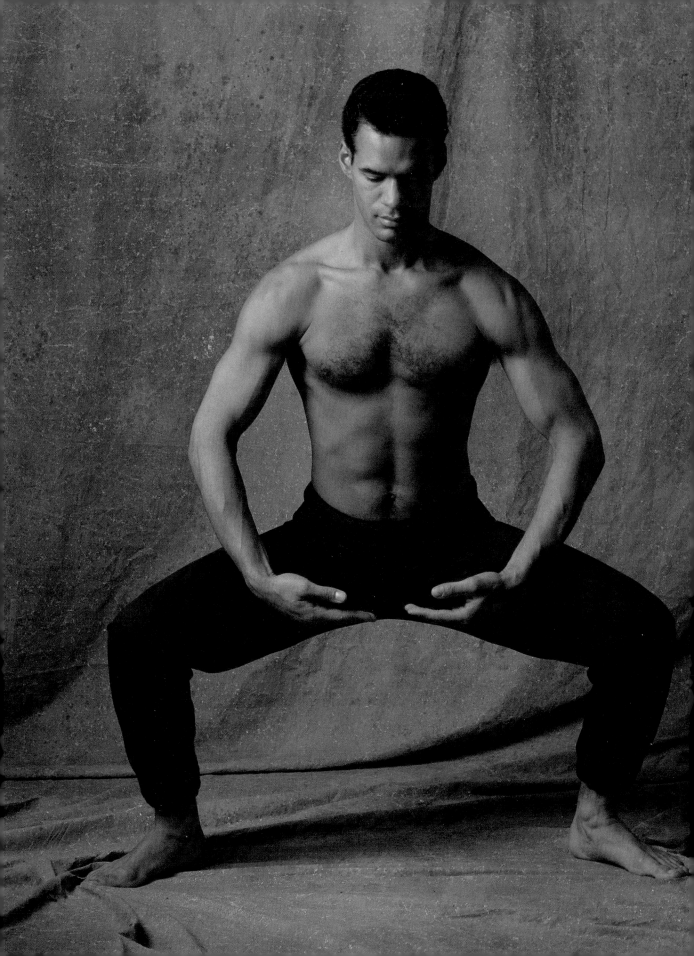

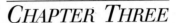

CHAPTER THREE

Concentration

*The elements of selective
attention — and how
to enhance them with Aikido*

Virtually any activity in which you want to excel requires concentration — the ability to bring all your faculties to bear on what you are doing. When you are concentrating totally, you are not conscious of how much effort you must make to accomplish your task: You simply do it. Total concentration is elusive; you can achieve it, paradoxically, only by *not* working on it directly. Instead, to develop this skill, you must learn to shift your attention from yourself to what is happening — or is about to happen — in your environment and pay attention to relevant cues only, disregarding all others. For this reason, sports psychologists use the phrase *selective attention* to refer to the ability to concentrate.

When you are first learning an activity, you must focus consciously on each component of it and inwardly monitor every aspect of completing it. Even such a straightforward activity as running initially requires being aware of your stride, heel placement, arm swing and other aspects of technique if you are to perform it efficiently.

As you acquire skill and experience, the need for this conscious attention to what you are doing diminishes. You begin to blend the various components of an activity, and the execution becomes automatic and harmonious. Performing at this level frees you to focus outward on the environment — for example, to monitor the conditions of a running track or to hear your fellow musicians in an orchestra — enabling you to cope effectively with variables. Once you have mastered your skill, focusing outward requires that you assume a state of consciousness that the poet William Wordsworth called a "wise passiveness." Swimmers describe this feeling as one of being pulled along by the water; runners sometimes explain the feeling as floating along in a race as passive observers, almost as if others were doing the work for them.

Once you have reached a certain level of skill, you will find that focusing closely on one or more components of the activity — whether you are running or playing a musical instrument — is likely to disrupt both your performance and your enjoyment of it. There are times, of course, when you want to focus deliberately on one aspect of an activity in order to perfect your technique — to work on your backhand in tennis, for example, or to practice your kick in a swimming stroke. Ultimately, when you put all the components together, you want the result to feel effortless.

Practicing an activity will, by its very nature, help enhance your concentration. Athletes have developed particular techniques to heighten their concentration in competition (these are covered in detail in Chapter Four). For building overall powers of concentration, one type of exercise that has proved highly effective is martial arts training because it requires that you do complex, ritualized routines and movements repeatedly until they become rhythmic, graceful and smooth.

Many of the exercises in this chapter are derived from a Japanese martial art called Aikido. Pronounced *eye-key-doe*, this term is translated as the "way for the harmony of spiritual energy." Perhaps more than any other martial art, Aikido requires that you relax in order to be aware of and blend in with every facet of your environment. You must remain alert to any threat and then respond automatically to avoid or meet the provocation. Practitioners often describe their optimal state of mind as outwardly passive and calm, but reflective of everything around them.

Rather than attempt to counter a direct blow, such as a punch, with a block and a counterpunch or kick, an Aikidoist allows the attacker to throw the punch or make the assault. In response, however, he moves his body in conjunction with the attacker's momentum, changing the thrust of the assault slightly to throw the attacker off balance. Aikidoists believe that by making use of the attackers' strength, their own strength is doubled.

In addition to using their skills for self-defense, Aikidoists strive for spiritual improvement. By blending the energies of the attacker with

A Guide to the Martial Arts

There are more than 300 different martial arts. Since most of them are known in the West only by their Oriental names, it is often difficult to distinguish them. Here is a list of some of the most popular forms:

◆ **JUDO** This Japanese form of self-defense utilizes various throws, grapples and strikes. Judo, or "gentle way," is a competitive sport and an official Olympic category.

◆ **JUJITSU** Meaning "gentle art," Jujitsu is often credited as the forerunner of both Aikido and Judo. Jujitsu employs kicking and striking with throwing and holding.

◆ **KARATE** This "empty hand" technique is associated by Westerners with brick and board breaking, either with bare hands or feet. However, Karate is actually not a uniform system of self-defense but a term that covers many styles, including a Korean version, at least two Okinawan forms, four Japanese styles, several Chinese varieties and numerous others.

◆ **KENDO** This is a Japanese "sword way" of fencing that is performed with bamboo swords. Participants usually wear protective head, chest and arm gear to avoid injury from the physical contact of the bamboo sticks.

◆ **KUNG FU** Meaning "skill," "task" or "work," this term refers to the Chinese martial arts in general, although most Kung fu schools teach Chinese boxing.

◆ **SUMO** Sumo, or "struggle," is a Japanese form of wrestling. Since the winner is the one who can force any part of his opponent's body other than his feet to touch the ground, the most successful Sumo wrestlers tend to be very heavy. Many weigh more than 400 pounds.

◆ **TAE KWON DO** This martial art is the Korean form of Karate, which is translated as the "ways of hands and feet." Tae kwon do, along with a Japanese system, is the most popular style of Karate taught in the United States.

---

the defender, Aikido movements promote harmony between the fighters, obscuring the distinction between them. Thus, Aikido is a technique for reconciliation. In Aikido, there are no winners or losers; it is not a competitive activity. Aikido also teaches that combat is ultimately senseless, since the victor today may very well be the loser tomorrow.

Training in the martial arts in general — and particularly in Aikido — can help you put other aspects of your life in better perspective. Some athletes, for instance, claim that martial arts training helps them avoid frustrations and emotional problems that they encounter in their competitive sports. Indeed, Aikido training has also been used effectively as a theoretical approach to psychotherapy.

Most of the routines that follow in this chapter are exercises adapted from Aikido techniques.

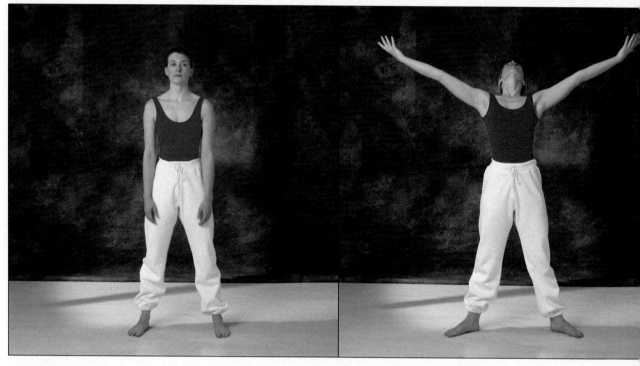

Aikido

The routines on these two pages and the ones that follow are adapted from Aikido. Although Aikido is a martial art, which usually requires two individuals, you can perform some Aikido movements alone, such as those shown on pages 69-93.

Aikidoists perform barefoot, a practice that is not only traditional but provides excellent traction as well. The best surface for working out is a wooden or carpeted floor, but you can also use an exercise mat. It is recommended that you wear loose-fitting, nonbinding clothing.

While performing the movements, do not become anxious or distracted by details. According to Aikido precepts, if you get caught up in your own thoughts or feelings, you will lose awareness of your surroundings and become vulnerable to attack. Remain calm using your mind as the surface of a pond, reflecting an image of everything around it.

Follow the movements slowly and carefully at first; you can speed up when you begin to feel comfortable with the various postures. Your goal should be to perform the Aikido without having to think about where to move next.

To perform Aikido routines, you should first relax through deep breathing. Stand erect with your feet apart and your hands at your sides *(above left)*. Draw your head back, your chest up and your arms out as you inhale deeply *(above)*. Exhale slowly and completely as you contract your body. Roll your head forward, bend your knees, bring your arms down and touch your fingertips together into a contracted position *(above right)*. Take a normal breath as you return to an erect but relaxed position *(opposite)*.

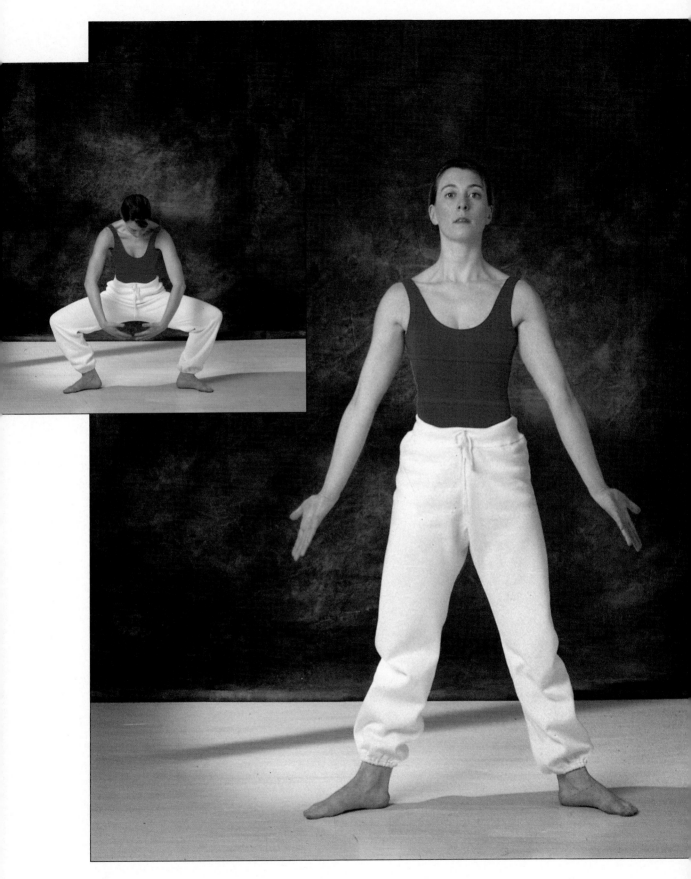

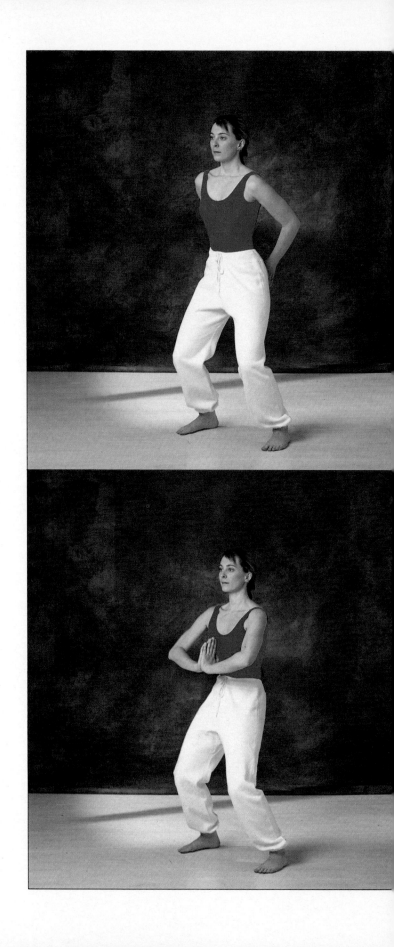

Ki Extension

Aikido masters draw power from their energy centers — *ki*, in Japanese. Stand in a relaxed position with your feet apart and your knees slightly bent. Press your hands into the small of your back *(far left)*. Still pressing your hands into your body, draw them around toward your stomach. Think of your hands as gathering strength from your center *(left)*. Capture that energy in your hands and bring them together *(below, far left)*. Throw your hands outward and gulp the air forcefully, then exhale *(below left)*.

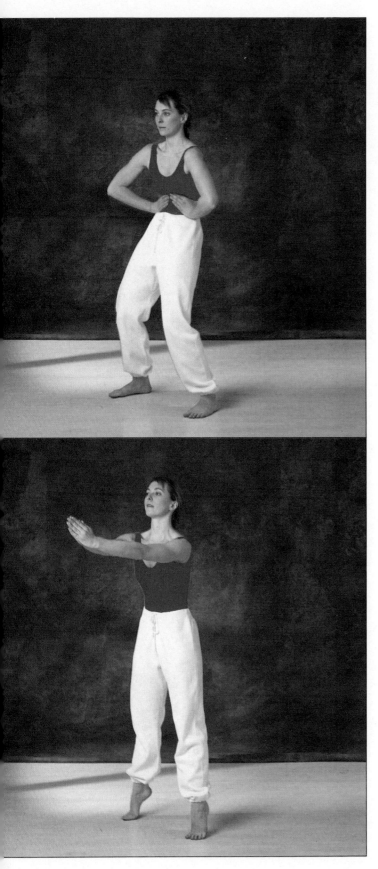

Moving Meditation

From an erect, relaxed position, extend your arms slightly and bend your knees so that you lower your center of gravity (1). Exhale as you bend over and press your hands against your shins. Inhale as you drag your hands slowly up your legs (2). Take a full breath as your hands reach the top of your chest (3). Hold your breath as you begin slapping down your body, from your chest to your ankles (4). With an explosive gesture and exhalation, thrust your hands toward the ceiling (5), and then inhale normally. Slowly exhale and round your body into a contracted position (6).

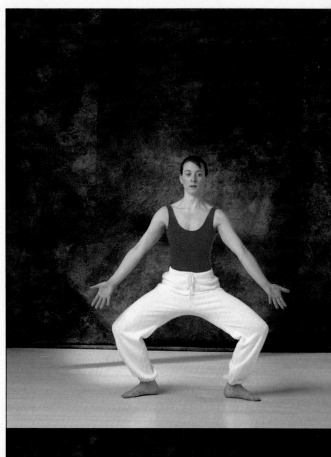

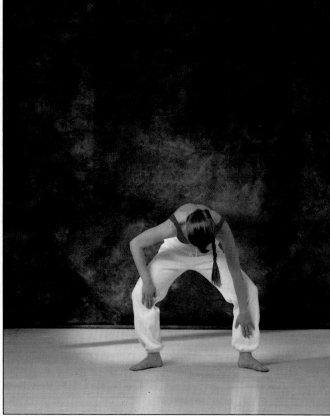

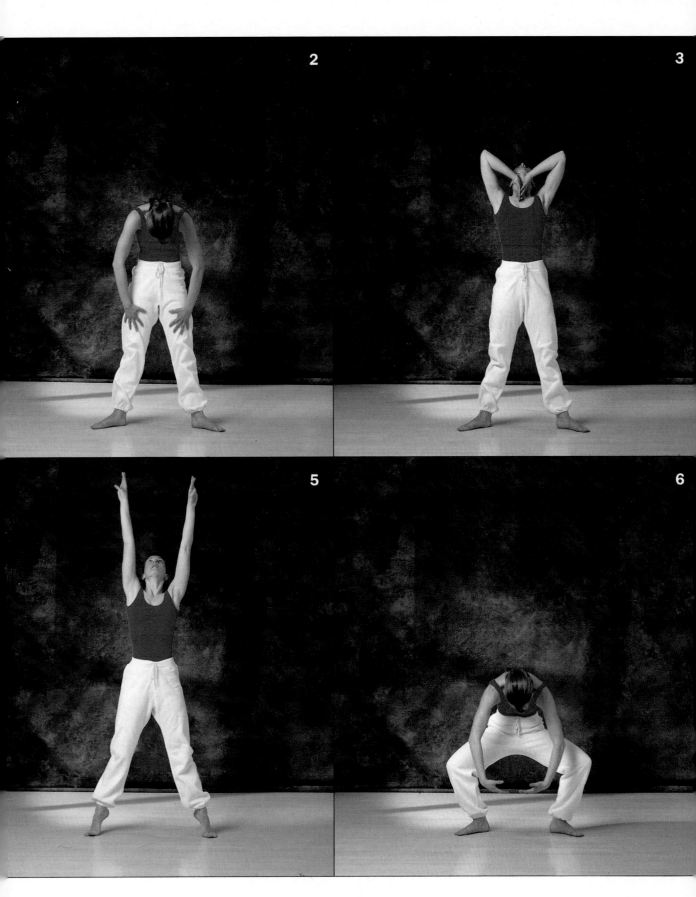

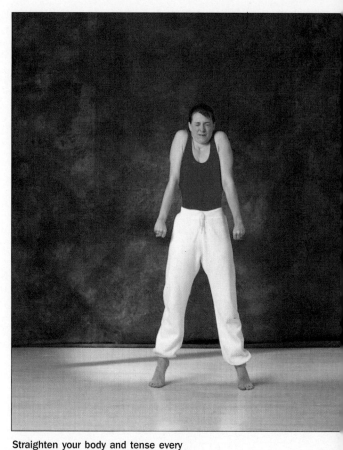

Straighten your body and tense every muscle. To center tension in your face, think of it as a hand that is balled up in a fist (7). Release that tension and relax into a grounded position with knees bent and arms spread at your sides (8). Lift your arms toward the ceiling and throw your head back as you rotate your body from the waist to the left (9). Perform a lunge to the left, dropping your arms slightly and extending them in front of you (10). Leading with your pelvis, draw back your body. Bring your right arm over your head, parallel to the floor (11).

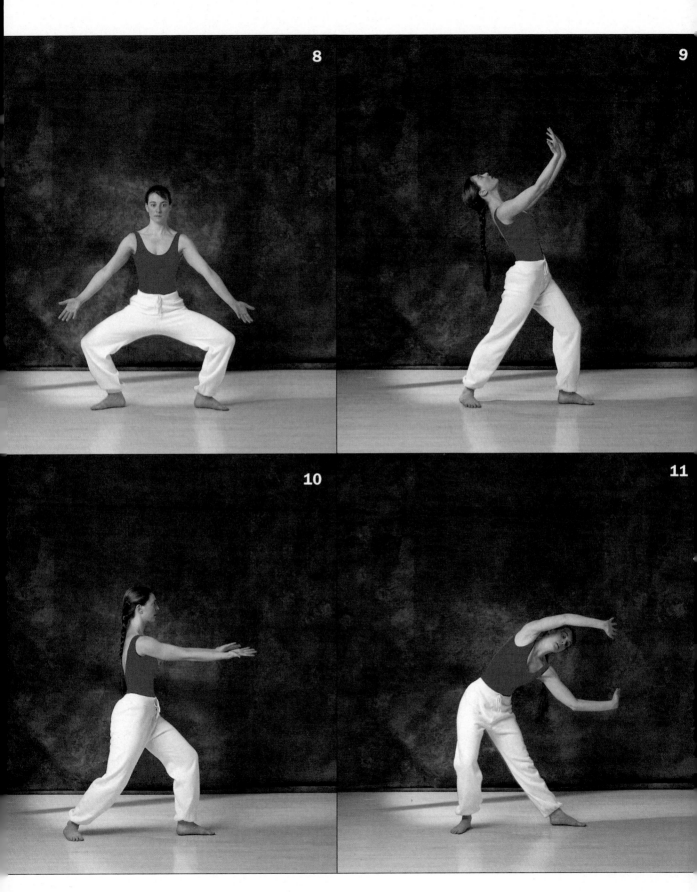

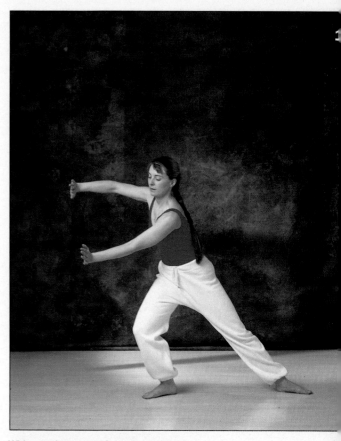

With your legs spread apart, sweep your arms to the right side as if you were pushing something (12). With your right hand, scoop inward toward your stomach to the left side (13). With your right arm, sweep outward and overhead, inscribing a large circle around your body. Allow your body to follow your arm, stretching to the right side (14), behind you (15) and to the left side (16).

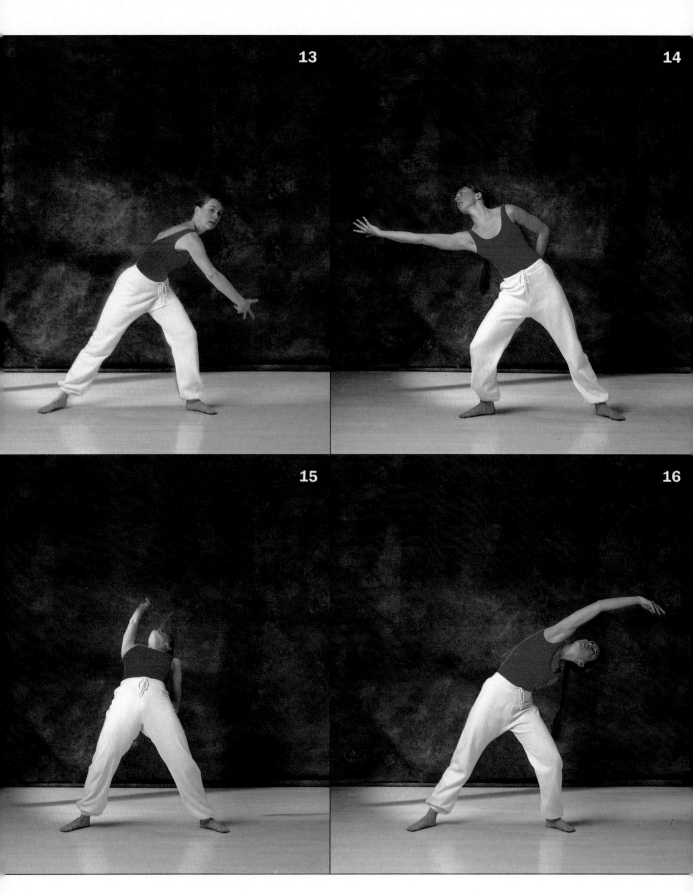

13

14

15

16

MOVING MEDITATION
(continued)

Continue spiraling to the right side (17). With a straight spine, bend at the hips and incline your torso to the right. Turn and face your whole body to the right, bringing your torso upright, inhaling and drawing energy back from your extended arm (18). Exhale and kick your left foot toward your right hand (19). Return to the grounded position and repeat the sequence from the beginning, this time following your left arm.

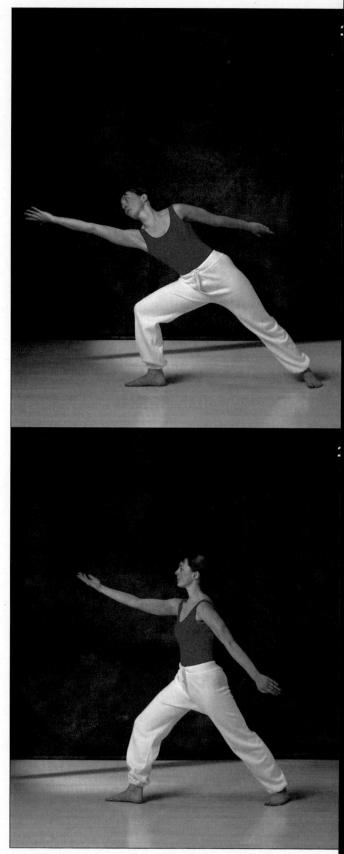

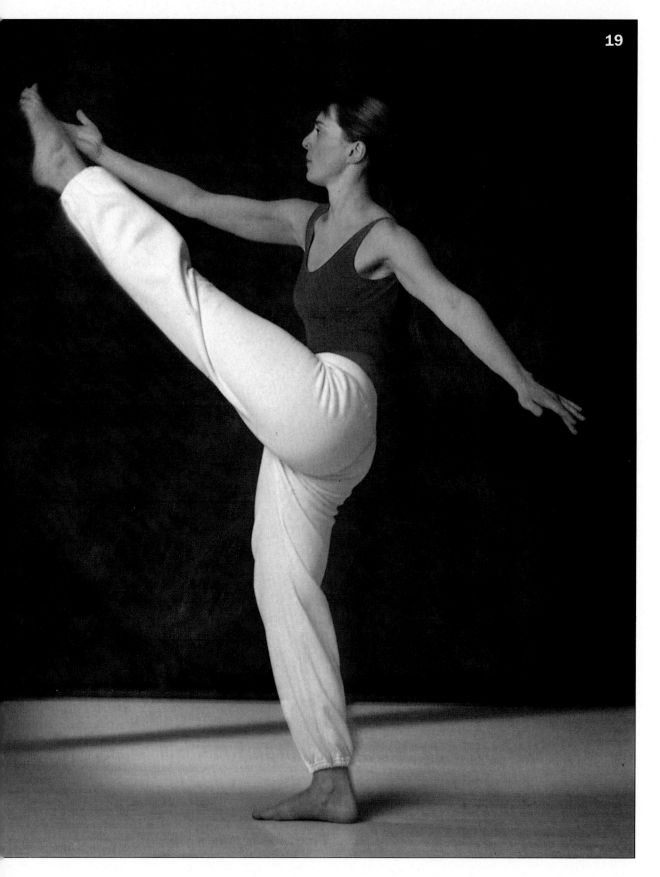

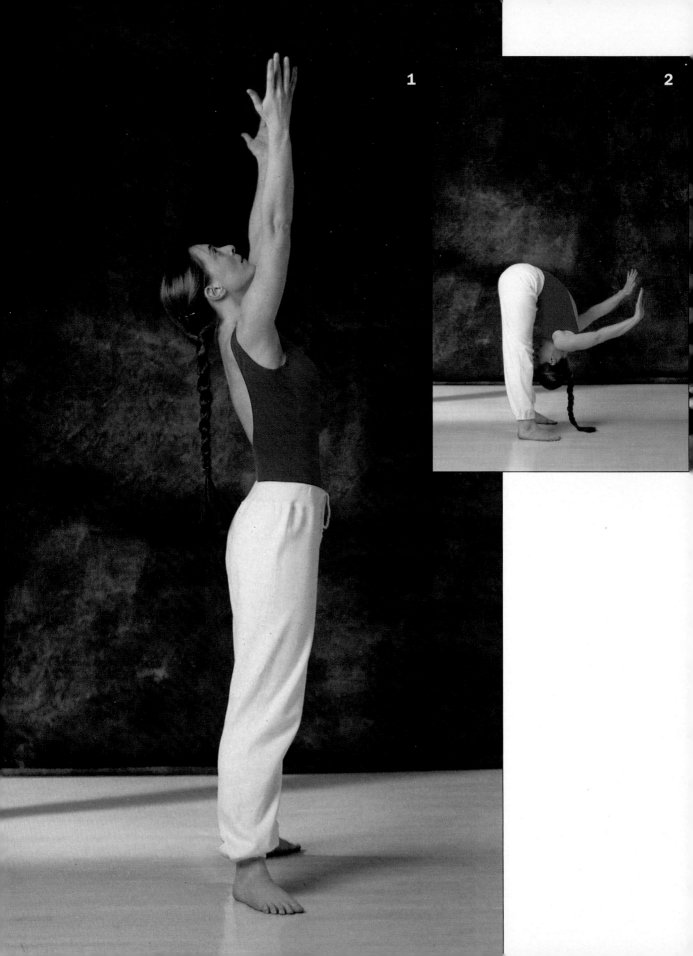

1

2

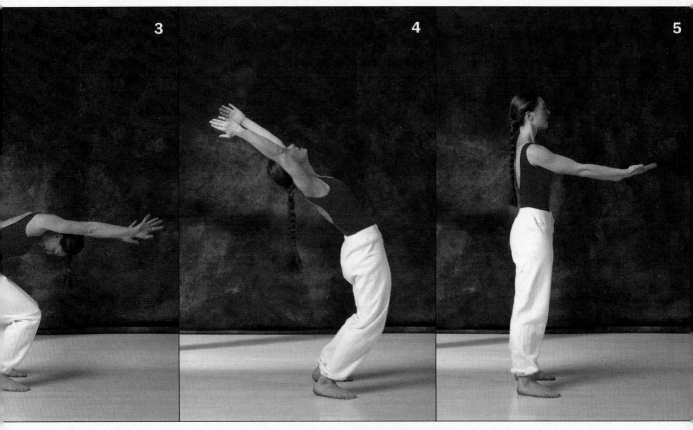

Moving Concentration

Stand erect and take a deep breath as you raise your arms, hands pointing toward the ceiling (1). Swing your arms down and as far back behind you as possible three times while you exhale and bend over progressively (2). Reverse the arm swings back and around in a circle and straighten your body, leading with your lower back (3). Continue moving past the erect position and extend your arms as far behind your head as they can go (4). Center your body, pressing your arms down parallel to the floor in front of you (5). Then press your arms down at your sides.

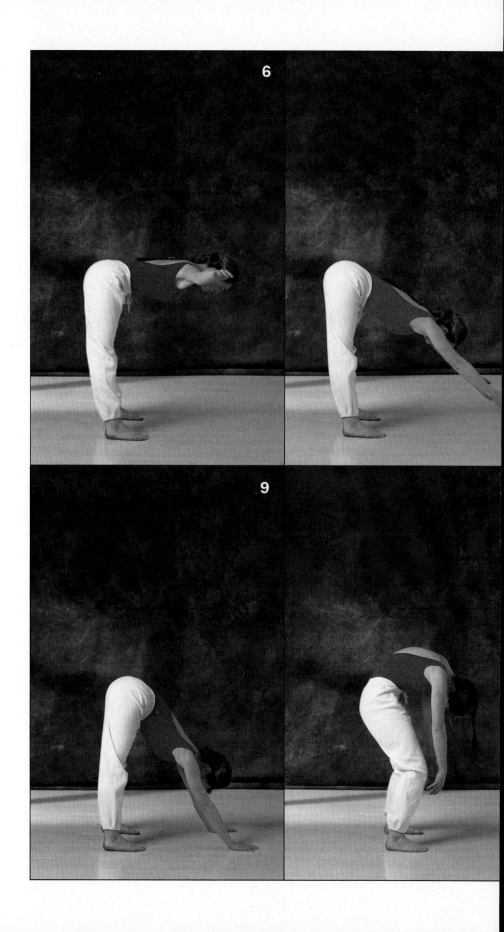

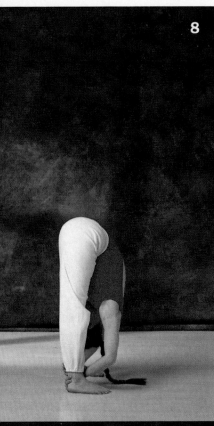

MOVING CONCENTRATION
(continued)

Inhale and bend at the waist, imagining your lower back as flooded with air. Keep your back flat as you extend your arms sideways (6). Reach your arms over your head and exhale, slowly releasing the air from your lower back and dropping your head toward the floor (7). Continue exhaling and deflating. Grip your ankles and try to straighten your knees, but do not force them (8). Inhale, lengthen your spine and extend your hands along the floor, forming a triangle (9). Continue inhaling and raise your hands off the floor. Exhale as you roll upward (10). Return to the grounded position (11).

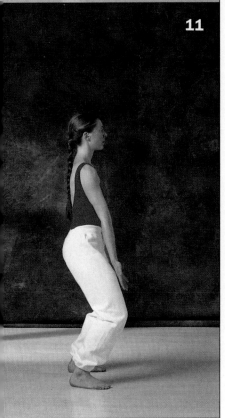

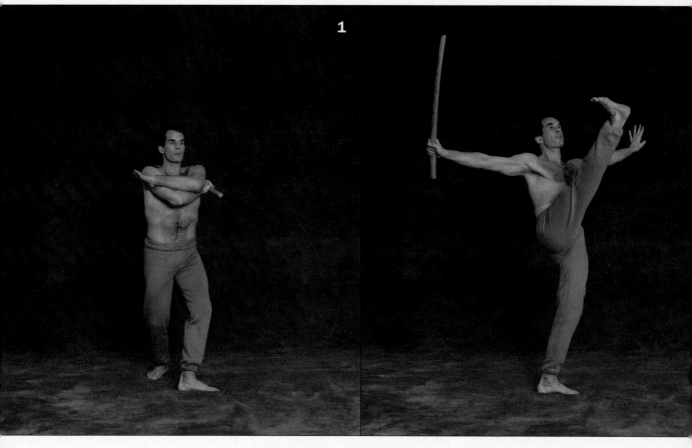

Sword Sequence

Many martial arts are known for defense methods that employ weapons. In Aikido, sword or staff routines are equally important to bare-handed techniques. The Aikido precepts of focusing and extension, in fact, become more apparent when you work with a sword and think of it as an extension of your body.

Many Aikido movements are the same whether you perform them with a wooden sword, a staff or no weapon at all. You can obtain the same benefits from the routine on these two pages and the following four, with or without a sword. You may even perform the exercise with two short sticks, one in each hand. Remember that the sequence shown here is not intended as a method of self-defense or attack.

If you do not observe safety precautions, you or another person in your range of motion can suffer serious injuries. When performing the sword sequence with a weapon of any sort, make sure that you are sufficiently clear of any objects or other persons.

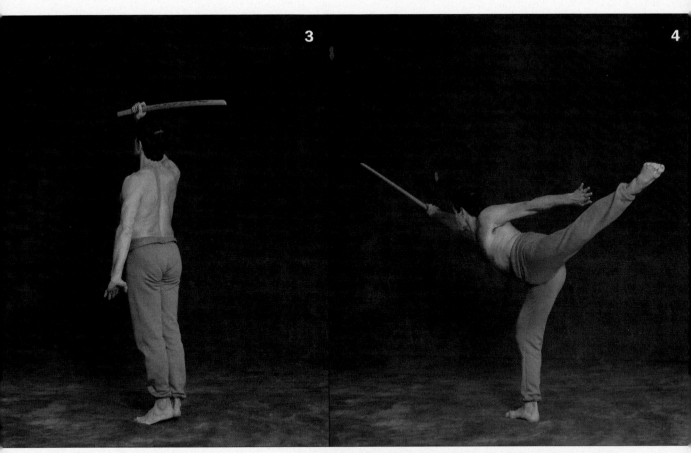

Stand erect and relaxed with a wooden sword or staff in your right hand. (If you are left-handed, hold the sword in your left hand and perform all right-handed directions with your left hand.) Take a half-step forward with your left foot and cross your arms over your chest (1). Exhale forcefully and kick your right foot up, thrusting your arms sideways (2). Return to the erect position, pivot 180 degrees and cock your sword arm (3). Exhale forcefully, bend forward and extend your sword arm and left foot (4).

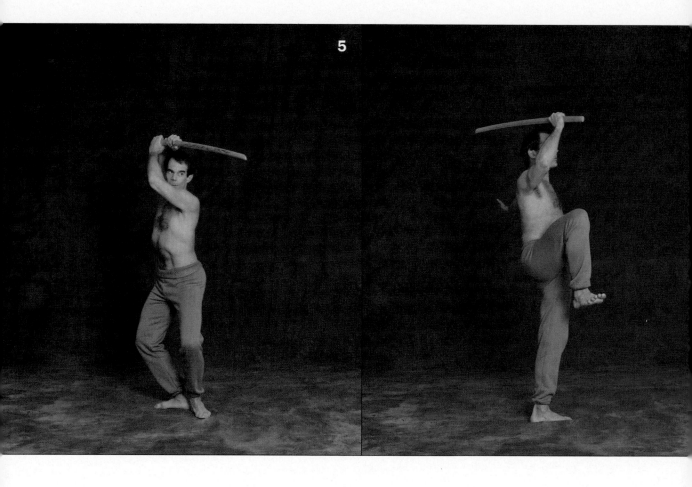

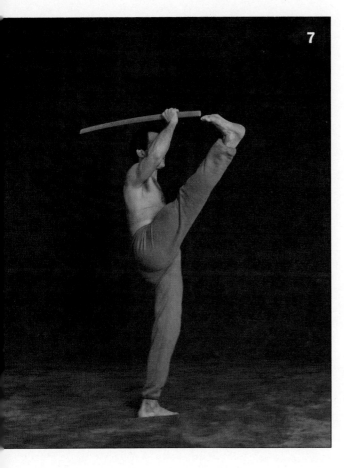

SWORD SEQUENCE
(continued)

Return to an erect position, pivot 90 degrees to the left and lift the sword over your right shoulder with both hands (5). Swing the sword over your head with your right hand; extend your left hand behind you and lift your right knee (6). Exhale and extend your right leg (7).

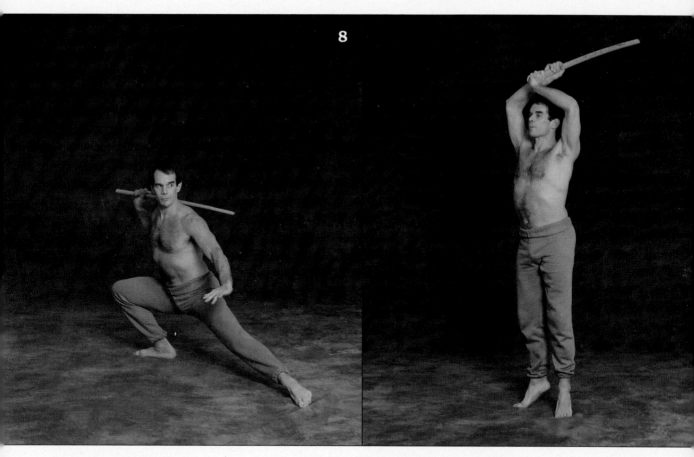

SWORD SEQUENCE
(continued)

Swing your right leg down behind you and
lower yourself with your right knee flexed
and most of your weight on your right
foot. Extend your left leg and lift the
sword so that it rests on your shoulder
(8). Take a deep breath and bring your
legs together, rise up on your toes and
draw the sword over your head with both
hands (9). Exhale forcefully and, extending the strength arising from your center
and through your arms, swing the sword
down in front, parallel to the floor (10).

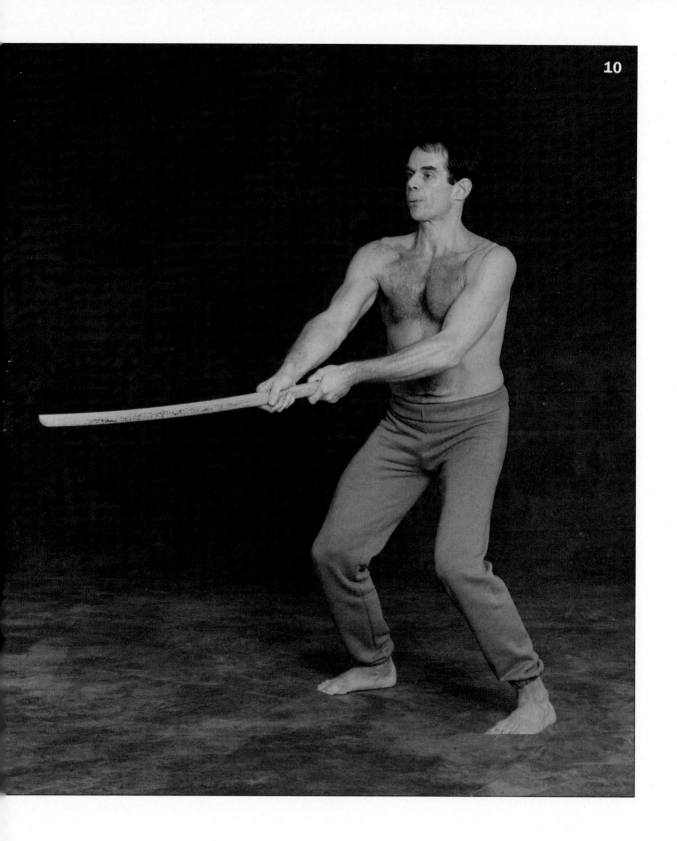

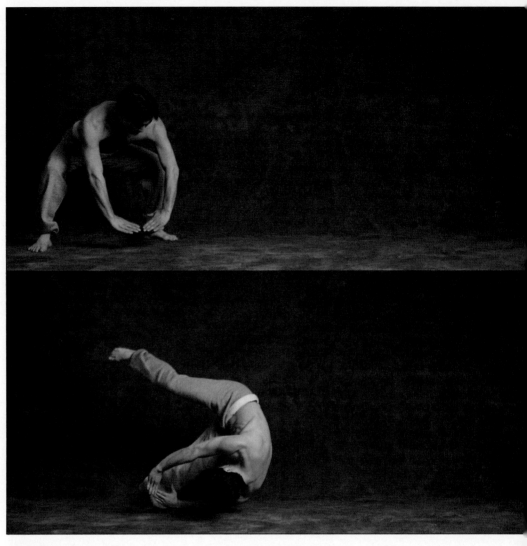

Rolls/1

Before performing Aikido with a partner, you should learn how to fall safely. The two basic safe falls are the front roll and the back roll, as shown on these two pages and the following two.

A roll is a technique in the self-defense arsenal. It is a way to absorb an impact or deflect a blow so that you can recover quickly and return to defend yourself. At the same time, rolls are part of a movement sequence that can help enhance agility and balance. If you feel yourself losing your balance, you should allow yourself to complete the fall. If you resist, you may become stiff and tense, which will result in a clumsy fall and increase your risk of injury.

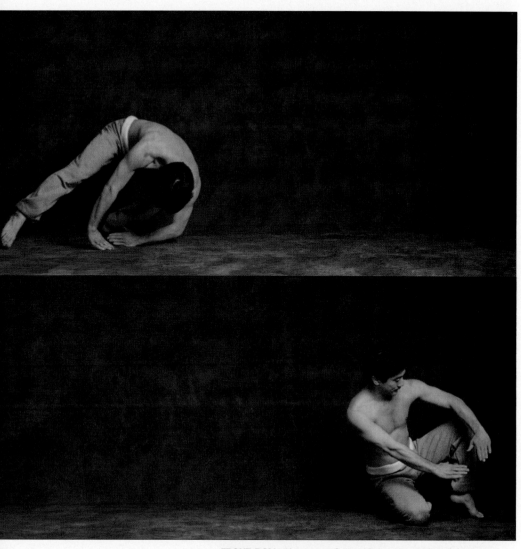

FRONT ROLL Keep your feet wide apart and bend down to roll on your left side *(top left)*. Making sure that your left arm is curved, not straight, push off with your right foot and roll over your shoulders *(top right)*. Turn your head to the side so that you will not roll over your head *(above left)*. Complete the roll, tucking your right leg under you *(above right)*, and stand up.

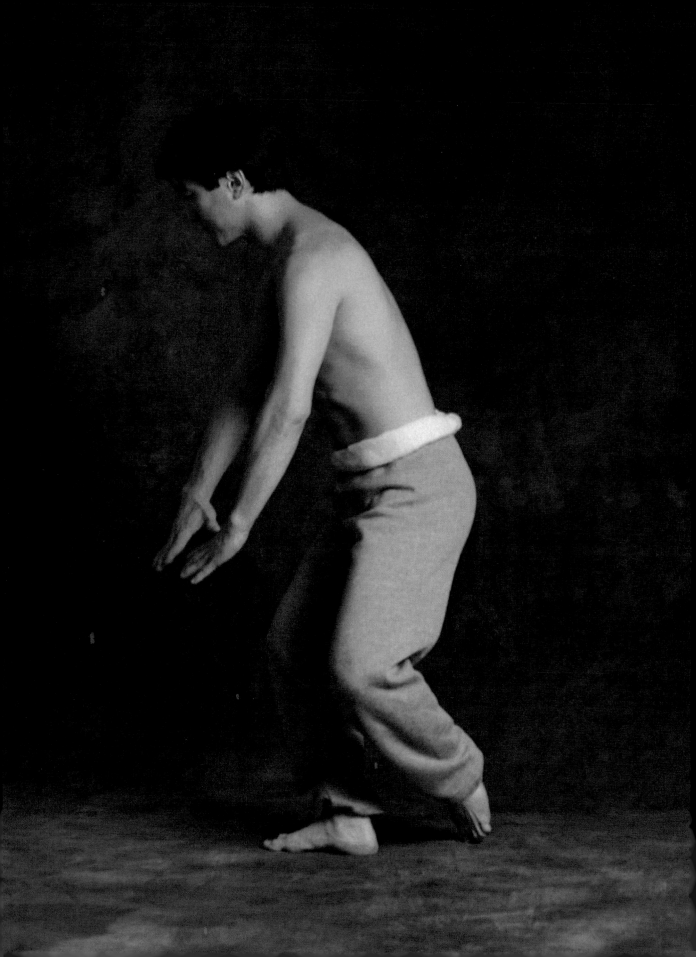

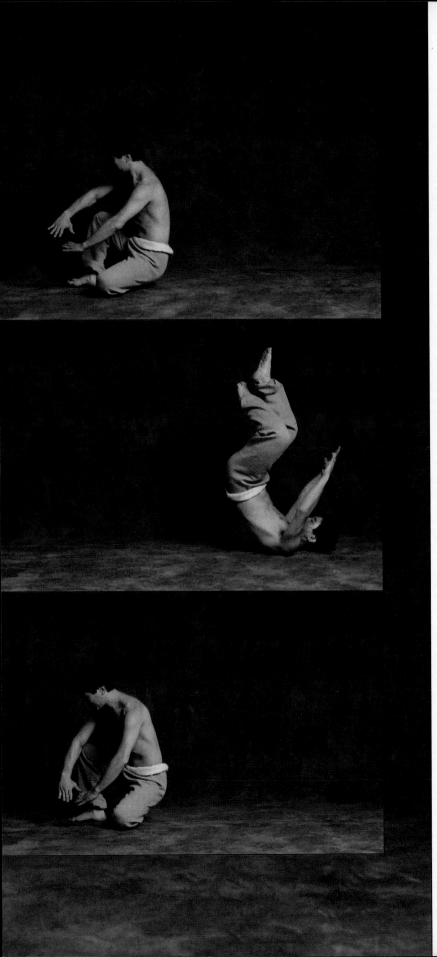

Rolls/2

BACK ROLL To start the backward roll, place the toe of your left foot behind your right *(far left)*. Fall back so that your left leg folds under your body but your right foot is still flat on the ground *(top left)*. Push with your right foot and roll on your right shoulder *(center left)*. Do not roll over your head, but use your momentum to reverse the backward roll and return to a crouch with your left leg tucked under you *(bottom left)*. Return to a standing position to complete the roll.

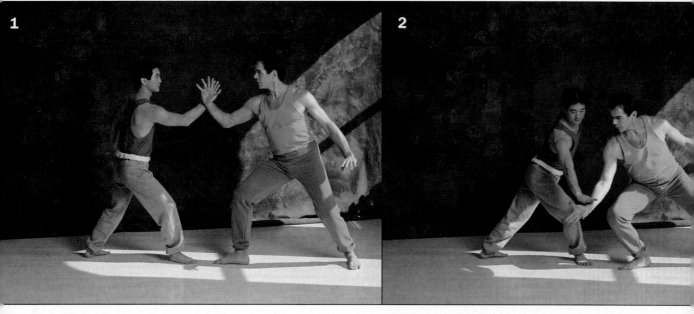

Partner Sequences

Although many martial arts routines can be practiced individually, the proper performance of a technique requires a partner. Although Aikido is devoted to peace, not conflict, the defender is prepared for the attacker's thrust. The defender must try to blend with the attacker physically and mentally so that their energies are combined. When that happens, the attacker's force is dissipated and the conflict is neutralized. At that point, the defender gains the advantage. He throws the attacker off balance so that the attacker makes a controlled fall, absorbing the impact of the throw.

In practice, the thrust of most attacks comes in a straight line, either from a punch, strike, grab or a kick. The Aikidoist transforms the linear force into a circular motion, dissipating its strength and leading the opponent's energy harmlessly aside.

Mastering the thousands of Aikido techniques requires consistent, long-term dedication. Also, perfecting most of these techniques necessitates formal training under an Aikido master, a person who has studied the forms and acquired the basic principles of universal harmony.

The techniques on these two pages and the following ten should not be considered comprehensive; nor are they intended as a substitute for working under a master's supervision. Practicing these routines can help strengthen your body and also sharpen your mind.

As with the Aikido exercises you perform alone, do the partner routines slowly and smoothly at first, building up speed and power as you become familiar with them.

When describing partner-blending routines in the martial arts, it is customary to use the terms *attacker* and *defender* to differentiate between opponents. This does not imply there is an aggressive confrontation. In the photographs that follow, partners are identified by their shirt colors for clarity. Perform each routine eight times — four times as the attacker and four times as the defender. Alternate attacks and defenses from the right side and the left side in order to feel comfortable in every position.

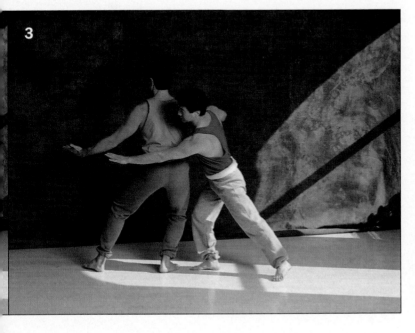

Ki Contact Exercise

Stand facing your partner. Position yourselves so that the backs of your hands cross when you both step forward with your right feet and extend your right arms (1). PURPLE: Try to grab green's right hand. GREEN: Lead purple's right hand down and across to your left side (2). PURPLE: Reach for green's left arm with your left hand. GREEN: Step around your opponent so that he is behind you. Maintain body contact with your right arms during the movement (3).

KI CONTACT EXERCISE
(continued)

GREEN: Center yourself in front of your opponent. PURPLE: Grab green's wrists from behind (4). GREEN: Lift up your right hand and pull down your left as purple twists to your left (5). Continue the rotational movement, turning your opponent around (6). Center purple directly in front and lower your arms so that he bends over backward into a back stretch (7). All your movements should begin from the waist.

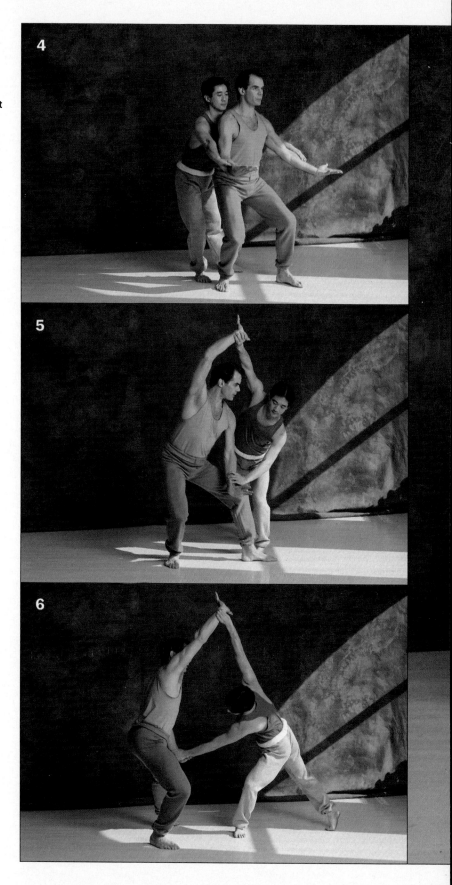

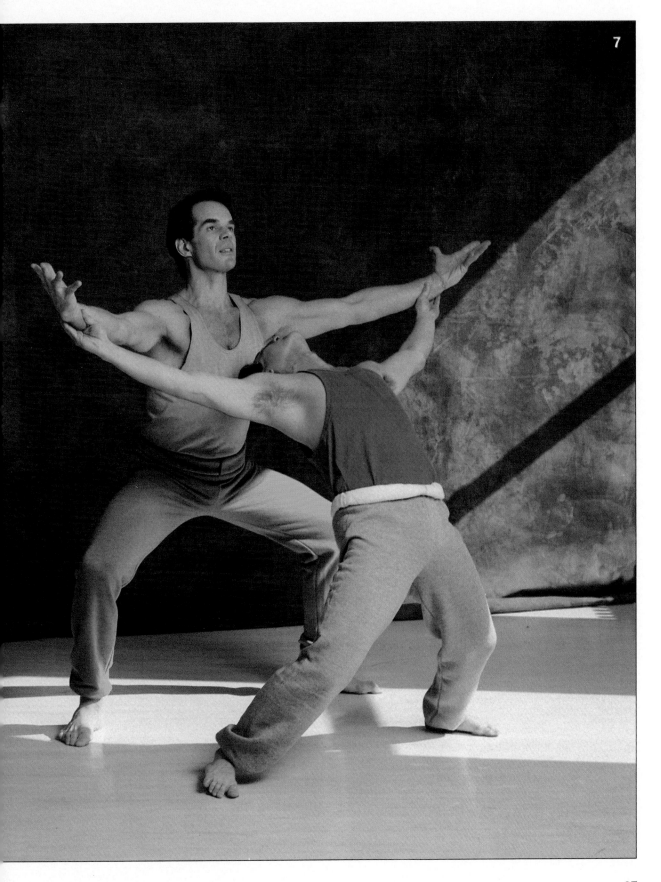

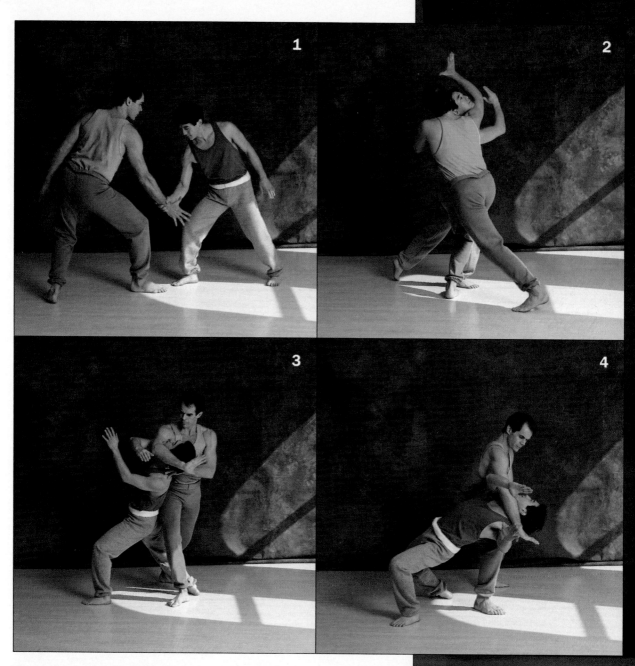

Rotational Throw

Resume the starting position facing each other, with right legs forward and bent slightly. PURPLE: Grasp green's right wrist (1). GREEN: Swing your arm down, around and up, leading purple's arm so that he loses his grip but maintains contact. Step forward and behind purple, locking your right arm under his chin (2). Place your left hand between purple's shoulders or on his neck and twist him to the right (3). Bring purple into a back stretch, being sure to support him firmly on your right knee and with your left hand on his back (4). As an optional throw, lower purple carefully toward the floor and, when you are both ready, release him (5), making sure that he does not land flat on his back. Using the techniques shown on pages 90-93, he should absorb the impact by rolling on his left arm and shoulder.

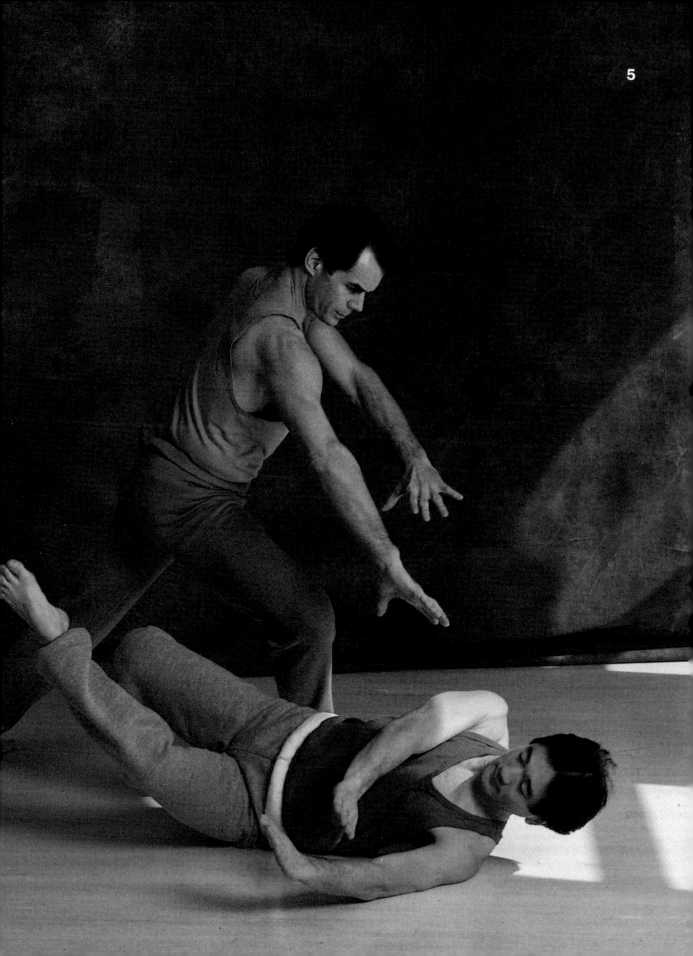

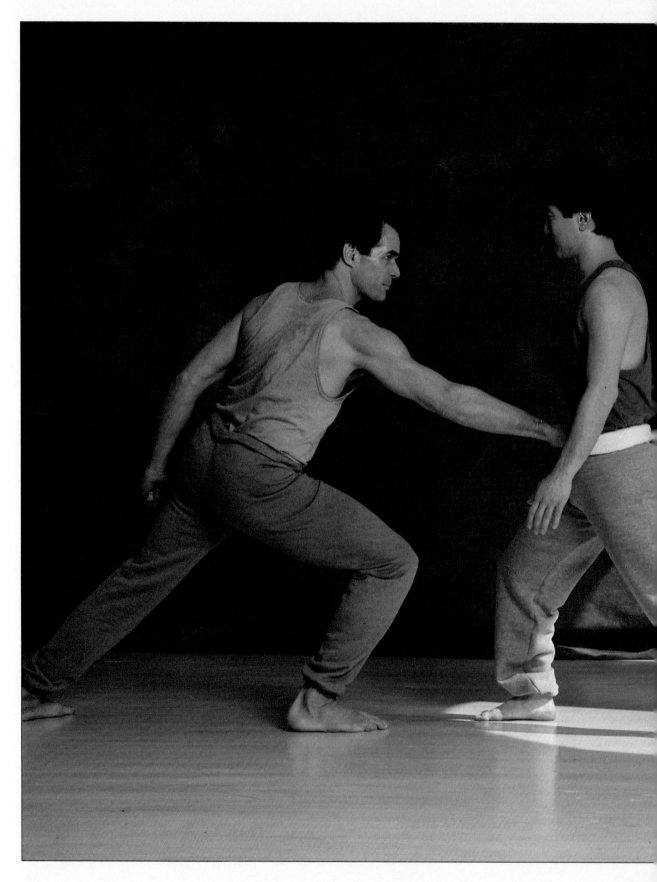

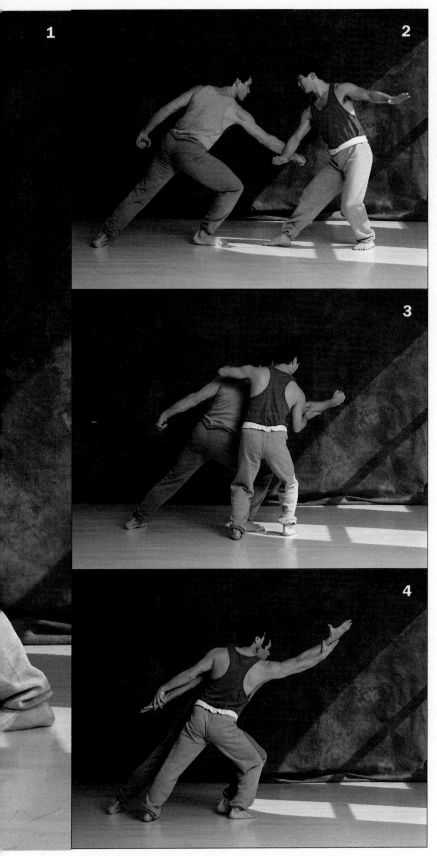

Center Walk

Start by facing each other in the same half-lunge position as in the two preceding sequences. GREEN: Place your right fist on purple's lower abdomen. PURPLE: Tighten your lower abdominal muscles and push green from your center by taking three forward steps (1). Then thrust aside green's right arm with yours (2). Step behind green (3) and extend your right arm with green's right arm, your left with his left so that your energies blend (4).

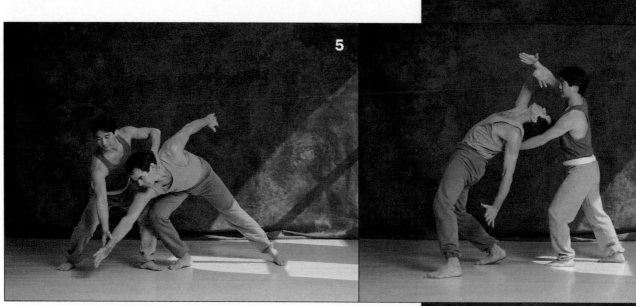

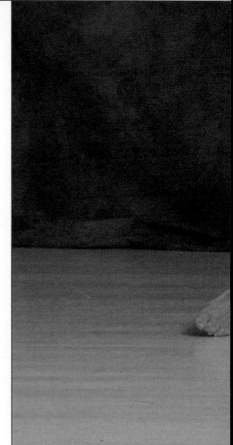

CENTER WALK *(Continued)*

PURPLE: Leading green's right arm downward, twist green's torso in a circular motion around to the right (5). Continue the circle and lead green's right arm over his head. Place your left hand in the middle of green's upper back to support him and draw him back for the stretch (6). As an optional throw, you may lead your partner farther back and, when you are both ready, release him (7). Your partner must not land flat on his back but land on either side, rolling so that his arm and shoulder absorb the impact.

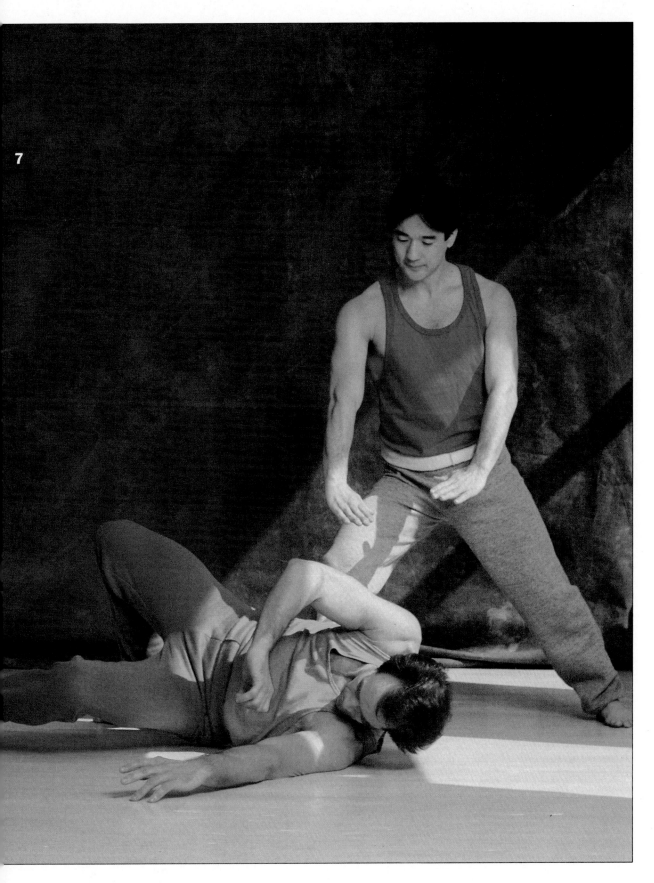

7

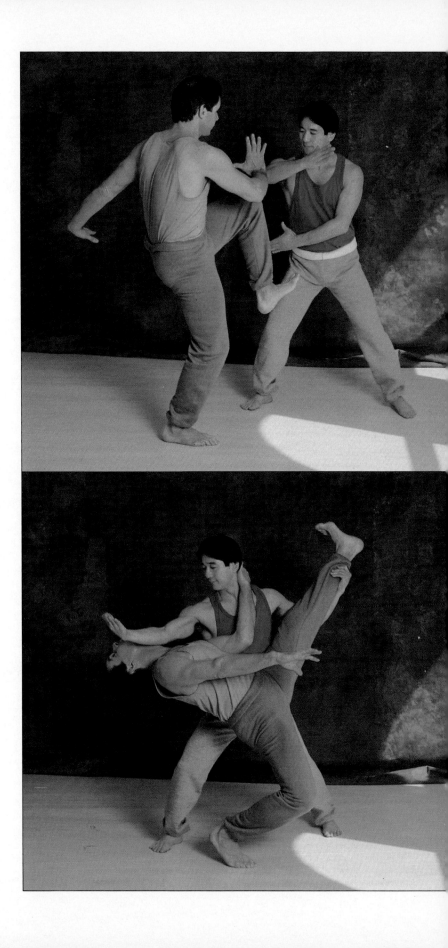

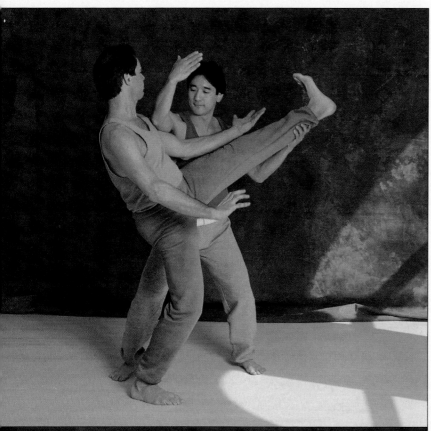

Kick to Center

Stand facing each other. GREEN: Lift your left leg to kick as purple prepares to move aside *(far left)*. PURPLE: As green completes the kick, move to his left, grip his left ankle and extend your right arm above and beyond green's face *(left)*. Hold green's extended foot in place and extend your right arm, stretching green backward. GREEN: Support yourself by holding onto purple's neck with your left hand *(bottom, far left)*. As an optional throw, lower your partner until you are both ready and then release him *(bottom left)*. Your partner must not land flat on his back but roll on one arm and shoulder to break his fall.

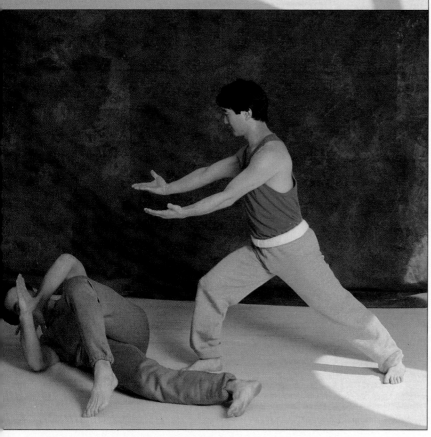

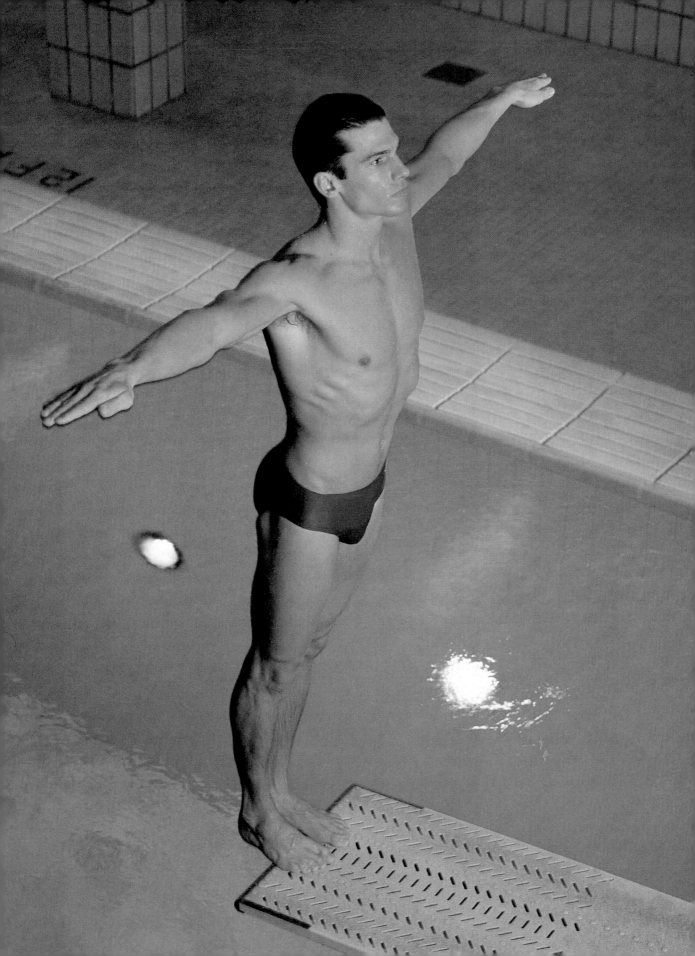

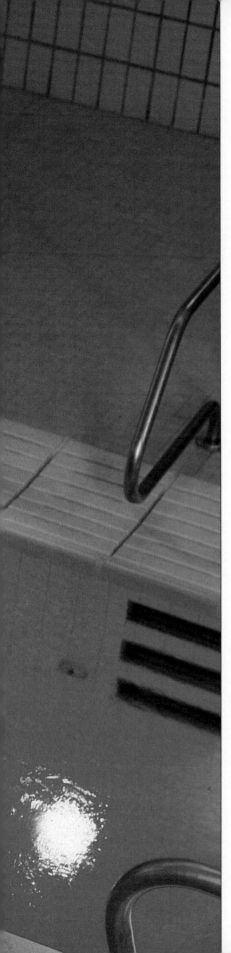

CHAPTER FOUR

Focusing for Sports

The mental tools for peak performance

I f you play any sport regularly, even as a weekend athlete, you are probably aware that mental factors can affect your performance significantly. You may have spent hours practicing until your tennis serve, your swimming stroke or your golf swing are absolutely right, yet during an actual game or competition, your technique can fail. You become anxious and tighten up; you make one slip, then another, even as you try harder. Upset and distracted, you find yourself losing to less talented players.

Most serious athletes acknowledge that psychological readiness is crucial for success in competition. Despite weeks or months of physical training, athletes who are not prepared mentally can usually perform brilliantly in practice, yet far below their potential during an actual event. One reason for such a lapse in performance is a lack of motivation, which results in inattention to the demands of the game. When this occurs, an athlete's mind is distracted and he does not extend himself. Just as undesirable as lacking motivation is being

107

overly conscious of the pressure to win, which typically produces anxiety about making an error. To compensate for this state of over-arousal, an athlete may rush to complete a play or a race, so that his timing and coordination are thrown off. His efforts will often be misdirected. Research into high-arousal/anxiety states indicates that attention narrows as arousal increases *(see box, page 109)*. While some athletes perform best at high arousal levels, and others are at their most effective at low levels, if a performer's arousal level exceeds his particular zone of optimal functioning, then his attention may focus too narrowly. The athlete tends to focus intently on the most obvious and direct stimuli, or he becomes overly concerned with minor details, screening out everything else, even those cues and behaviors that could benefit his performance. Furthermore, the greater the anxiety, the more likely his concentration will be shattered by distractions — from opponents, from spectators, from playing conditions, or even from his own thoughts.

A number of studies and individual reports from elite athletes suggest that it is not the absence of anxiety that leads to consistently superior performances, since almost all athletes experience anxiety before competition. Rather, the successful athlete has learned how to maintain his arousal level within a certain optimal zone and to channel the energy that the anxiety generates constructively.

According to sports psychologists, the ability to do this depends on your being able to adjust your attentional focus. When you are focusing your attention properly, the flow of information from your environment is processed by your mind unconsciously. You sort out what is useful from what is irrelevant and distracting automatically and without having to think.

You must adjust your attentional focus according to the type of activity you are engaged in. In sports that involve single concentrated tasks — such as hitting a golf ball, shooting at a target or kicking a field goal — your breadth of attention has to be narrow: You are focusing on one action or on a small area of your environment. Team sports, on the other hand, call for a broad focus, one that requires you to be aware of teammates, opponents, their positions and the action taking place on a field. Most team sports require the ability to shift between narrow and broad focusing, much like a camera's zoom lens. A basketball player, for example, needs a broad focus while pressing the opponents' basket with his teammates. When the ball is passed to him and he brakes to make a shot, he must suddenly tighten his focus onto the basket.

Another aspect of focusing is shifting between an internal and an external focus. For some activities, particularly endurance sports, the focus is often internal. A marathon runner, for instance, will frequently monitor his body for fatigue and fluid depletion while paying only periodic attention to his surroundings. Most sports and games, however, demand an ability to shift mentally between the self and what is happening — or about to happen — in the environment.

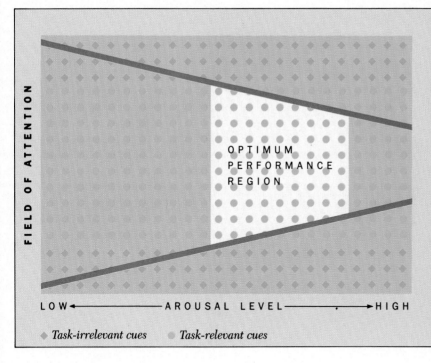

FIELD OF ATTENTION

OPTIMUM
PERFORMANCE
REGION

LOW ← —— AROUSAL LEVEL —— · → HIGH

◆ Task-irrelevant cues   ● Task-relevant cues

Focusing and Arousal

Any stimulus that you need to focus your attention on in order to accomplish your goal is called a task-relevant cue; stimuli that do not contribute to this end are task-irrelevant.

Researchers have found that as an athlete's arousal level rises, there is a resultant narrowing in perception and focus. This is good when the athlete eliminates task-irrelevant cues and his performance improves. But if arousal continues to rise, the athlete's attention can narrow until he excludes task-relevant cues, as when an anxious football quarterback overlooks peripheral receivers. Most people display this narrowing in attention, but whether they can keep it in a range for optimal performance depends on their experience and ability to focus.

Athletes who have developed their focusing ability have sometimes reported a sense of the action's slowing down or appearing larger than life, enabling them to perform this sorting process more effectively. Athletes have also reported shifts in alertness, having sharpened vision and hearing, and seemingly being able to anticipate where an action will occur. Such a state of mind also allows the athlete to more easily refocus after making an error or allowing a lapse in concentration.

Sports psychologists and athletes themselves have uncovered a number of techniques and exercises to help improve their focusing skills. The most effective of these are presented on the following pages, in the order that you would apply them in a performance situation. Not all of the methods will be appropriate to the sport or recreational activity of your choice, but you will benefit even if you employ only a few of them.

One of the best ways to find out which methods work for you is to keep a daily log. Keep track of how you feel; whether your focus is primarily internal or external, narrow or broad; and what mental training techniques you are using. In time, you will be able to determine which techniques work best to improve your focus. As you become more proficient at adjusting your focus, it becomes correspondingly less likely that you will worry or get distracted. And that, in turn, gives you a far better chance of performing consistently at your best.

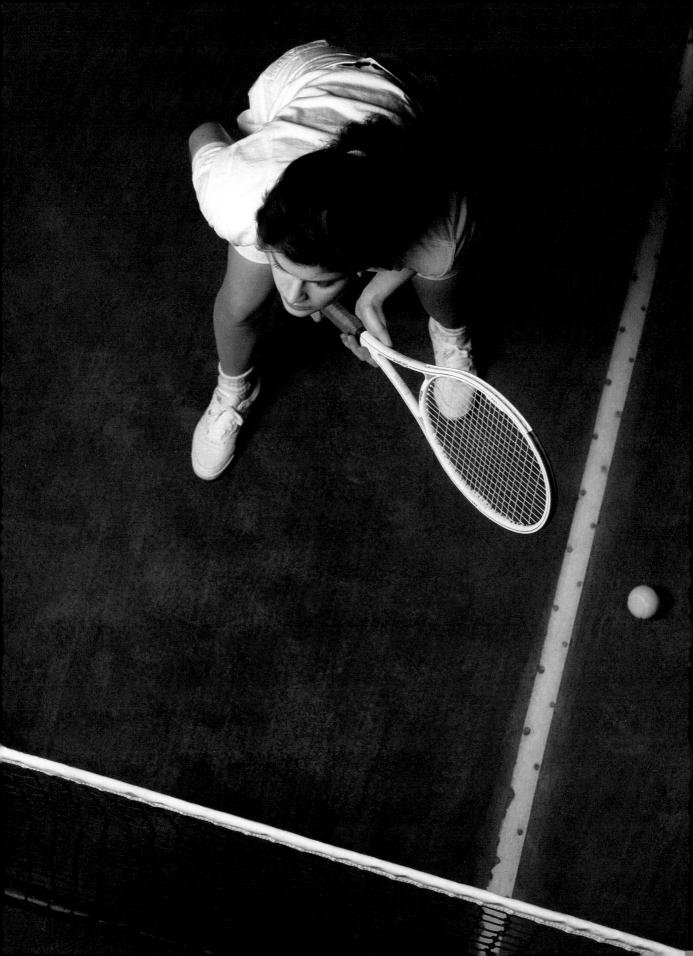

Previewing

Before a game or an event begins, you can mentally rehearse strategies, plays and specific skills that you will use. If you are a tennis player, for instance, start by visualizing yourself on the court. Think of your opponent's traits — for example, perhaps he has a weak backhand and he tires easily. Then visualize actually playing tennis against him, making him run in the backcourt. Hit your hardest drives to his backhand, then rush the net. As described on pages 18-19, visualize your play in "real time"; that is, rehearse your mental game at the same pace or speed it would be played in actual performance.

Every sport can be analyzed in this fashion and played mentally. If you are a golfer, preview the course in your mind and plan how you will hit the ball from various tees. If you are on a team, you can practice every conceivable play mentally. If you are guarding a goal or basket, visualize all the possible ways that the goal can be approached and how to guard it successfully. A gymnast or skater might rehearse how he or she would recover from a fall gracefully. Or if there is any skill you have particular difficulty with, imagine yourself performing it through every point at which an error or other problem might occur.

Relaxing

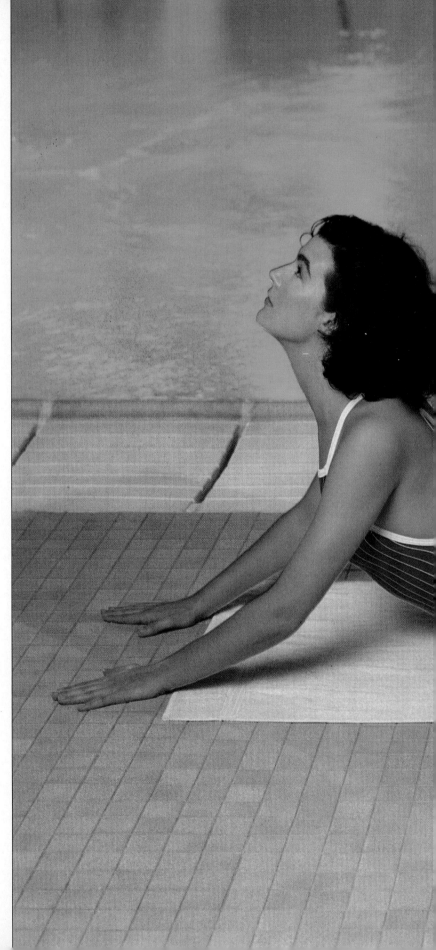

Another stage of preperformance readiness is becoming relaxed mentally and physically. Although a certain degree of arousal is necessary to perform at your optimum level, overarousal generated by anxiety results in nervousness and muscular tension. When one muscle or muscle group becomes tense, its opposing muscle group also contracts, leading to a tight double-pull on the joint the muscle is attached to. This double-pull can almost paralyze a person, causing an athlete to freeze up at the start of a performance. More often, muscular tension leads to an inability to perform skilled movements smoothly.

Relaxation techniques are useful for reducing both nervous anxiety and muscular tension. These techniques are of two categories: "mind to muscle" and "muscle to mind." Both are equally effective. Mind to muscle relaxation includes concentrating on deep abdominal breathing *(see pages 26-31)*. By focusing your attention on the calming effects of deep and steady breathing, you quiet your nervousness and reduce muscle tension.

Performing stretches to release muscular contractions, an example of muscle to mind relaxation, also has a calming effect. Many muscle stretches are involved in Yoga postures, which have been shown to reduce both muscular as well as psychological tension. Stretching one muscle will not relax another, however. You must slowly extend the muscle or muscle group that is tense and hold that position for at least 20 seconds, then repeat.

Often pregame anxiety produces tension in specific areas of your body. For example, a common tension response is to clench your jaws. Some athletes have found yawning relaxes their jaw muscles.

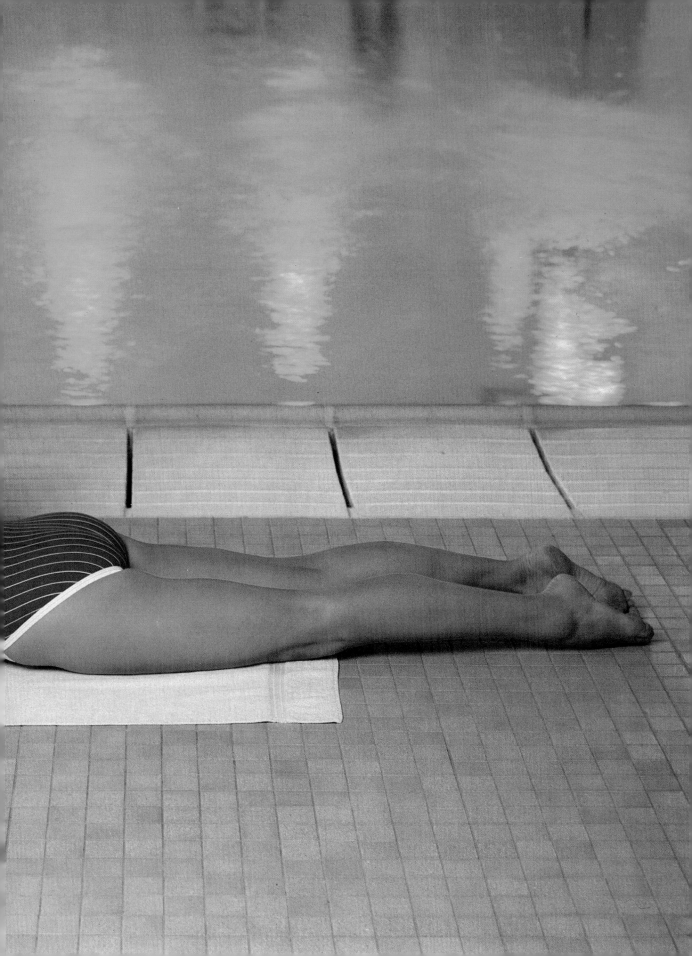

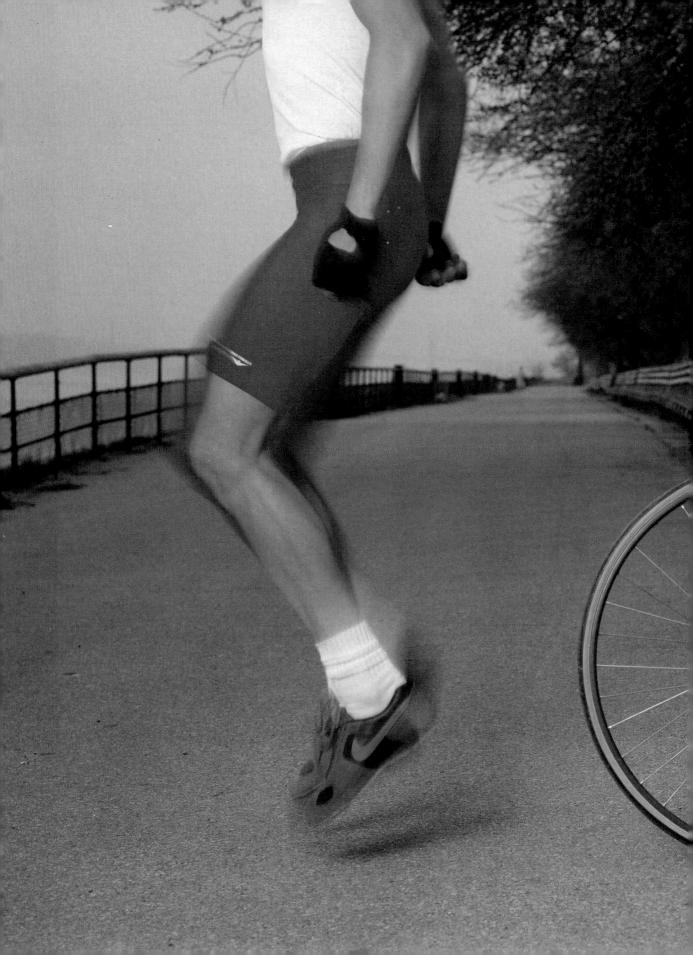

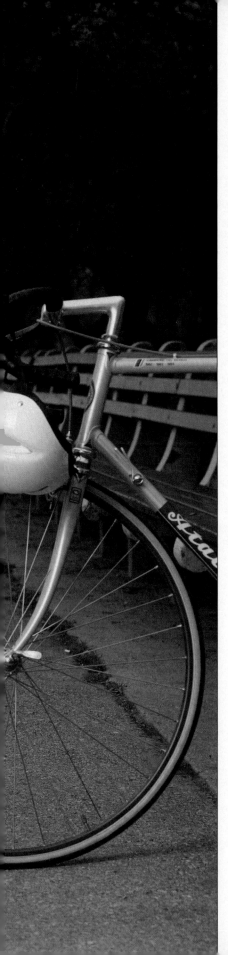

Activating

It is not uncommon for athletes to begin a game or an event feeling underenergized. An athlete in this low-arousal state may feel sluggish, unenthusiastic and easily distracted. Often this state is associated with a lackadaisical attitude about performance, as well as a poor sense of timing and anticipation during play. You can override these symptoms through activation techniques.

One of the easiest methods is simply to increase your respiration rate. Just as slow, deep breathing can calm and relax you, short, quick breathing is arousing physiologically, because it increases your heart rate and your circulation.

Another technique is to jump up and down or run in place while pumping your arms. This is one of the best ways to get your circulation moving. You can also think thoughts that trigger energetic emotions — thoughts of winning, of performing a particular play or maneuver well or of meeting an opponent in a challenging one-on-one encounter. The point is to create an image in your mind — symbolizing power, force or energy — that is not only positive but stirring.

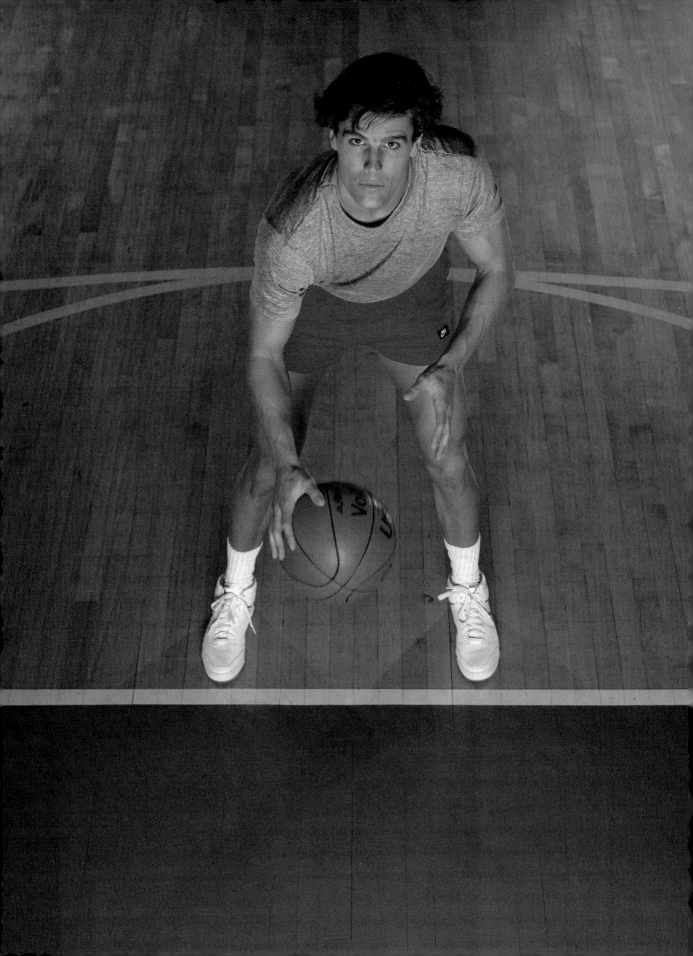

Using Rituals

During competition, many athletes perform rituals that do not contribute directly to their performance or to the actual game. Basketball players, for example, frequently bounce the ball several times before a free-throw shot; baseball players tap their shoes with a bat before hitting; pitchers massage the ball; tennis players often adjust their racquet strings before an important serve. These rituals are actually important techniques to help develop the right arousal level, maintain attentional focus and eliminate distractions.

Rituals often begin long before the competition. An athlete may eat special foods or wear a particular piece of clothing — habits that may be seen as mere superstition, but that often provide the athlete with a very real sense of security as the unknowns of competition approach.

In a game or an event, when lapses in concentration and in performance occur, you can regain control by taking the time to perform a ritual methodically. The action becomes an automatic relaxation and centering cue. Rituals also have a psychological effect on your opponent. When a batter, for instance, is forced to wait for the pitcher to perform his ritual of cocking his hat or scraping the ground, his anxiety and tension rise, making it more difficult for him to concentrate on the pitch.

Visualizing

J ust before performing an activity that requires skill, you should take a few moments to rehearse it mentally, step by step and in every detail. Visualizing each step clears the mind, eliminates distractions and concentrates your attention on performance.

For example, consider a track athlete who is about to run the high hurdles, an event that requires speed, agility and timing. As the hurdler settles into the starting blocks, he visualizes each stride toward the first hurdle. Leading with the right foot, the athlete may plan eight steps to the takeoff point seven feet in front of the first hurdle. It is crucial that the imagery contain movement rather than static techniques or positions, and it must be detailed. This apparently results in the sense of slow motion experienced by many athletes who perform complex tasks. Research indicates that successful athletes visualize their actions within milliseconds of the time of actual performance. For instance, a gymnast who visualizes an exercise routine takes the same amount of time imagining the performance as the event itself.

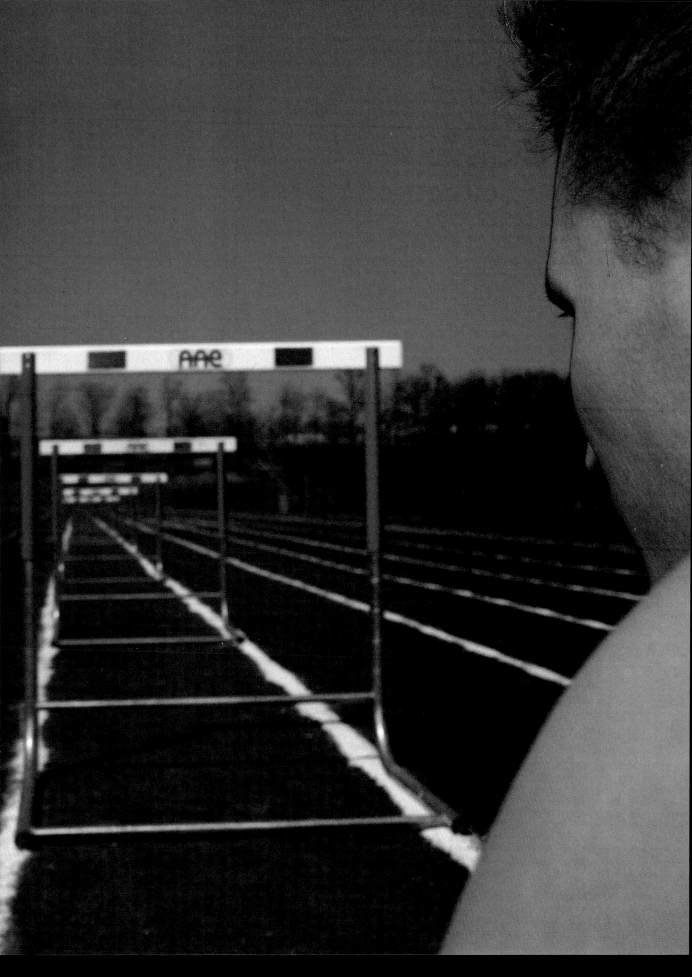

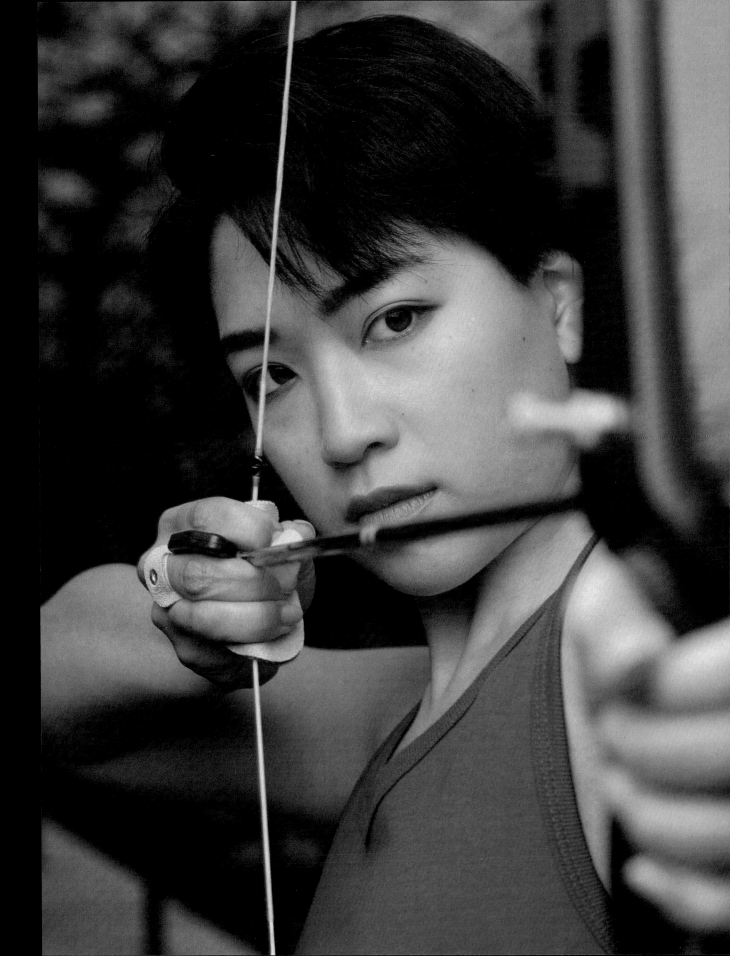

Focusing

Any action requiring exceptional muscular control — sinking a golf putt, shooting at a target, aiming a bowling ball, balancing on a high beam — demands the utmost concentration. Yet an athlete in this situation is often too aroused and can become highly sensitive to distractions. Some are internal physical sensations, such as a dry mouth, muscle tightness and slight nausea. Other distractions, such as audience noises or weather conditions, are external. In either case, consciously thinking about these distractions interferes invariably with the athlete's ability to concentrate.

In addition to rehearsing your performance mentally, you can ignore these distractions by narrowing your attentional focus, locking it on only the most relevant cues. An archer, for example, might begin by assessing wind, lighting conditions and other factors affecting the flight of the arrow. But at the moment before shooting, her concentration focuses on the target. Similarly, a golfer may scrutinize the conditions of a putting green, but he will focus his attention eventually on both the ball and the cup to make the putt. Some psychologists and athletes refer to this style of focusing as "hard eyes." When concentration is undisturbed, the athlete can often see the target with crystal clarity, as if it were larger than life.

Shifting Focus

In events that last any appreciable length of time, being able to adjust your attention over the duration of the action is essential to performing well. In sports that are physiologically demanding, an athlete should monitor his body, checking for fatigue, muscle tightness, energy states and breathing patterns along with mental responses such as confidence and anxiety levels. If, for example, an athlete notices that his jaw or fists are clenched, this should serve as a signal for him to relax. This self-monitoring is really a kind of internal focusing that sports psychologists refer to as association.

Endurance sports, such as long-distance running and swimming, call for dissociation — a tuning-out process that is akin to daydreaming. Whether you are jogging for recreation or running a marathon, dissociation can help stem boredom and will also shift your attention away from the discomfort of running.

Successful athletes have the ability to associate and dissociate as well as direct attention externally to assess the competitive environment. In a long-distance race, there will be times when you simply want to maintain a steady pace, which is a good time to dissociate. Periodically, though, you should direct your mind to monitor a sequence that might include assessing ground and weather conditions, the position of other racers, changes in their pace and your own energy level; then you can narrow your attention to make any necessary adjustments.

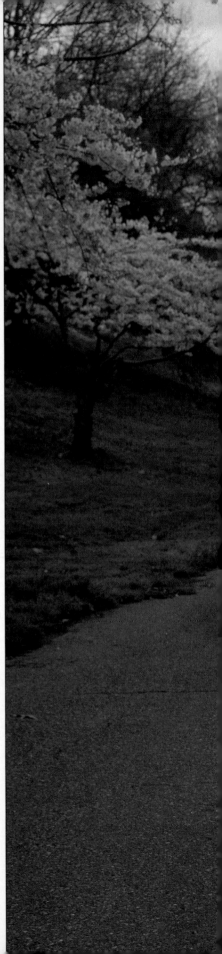

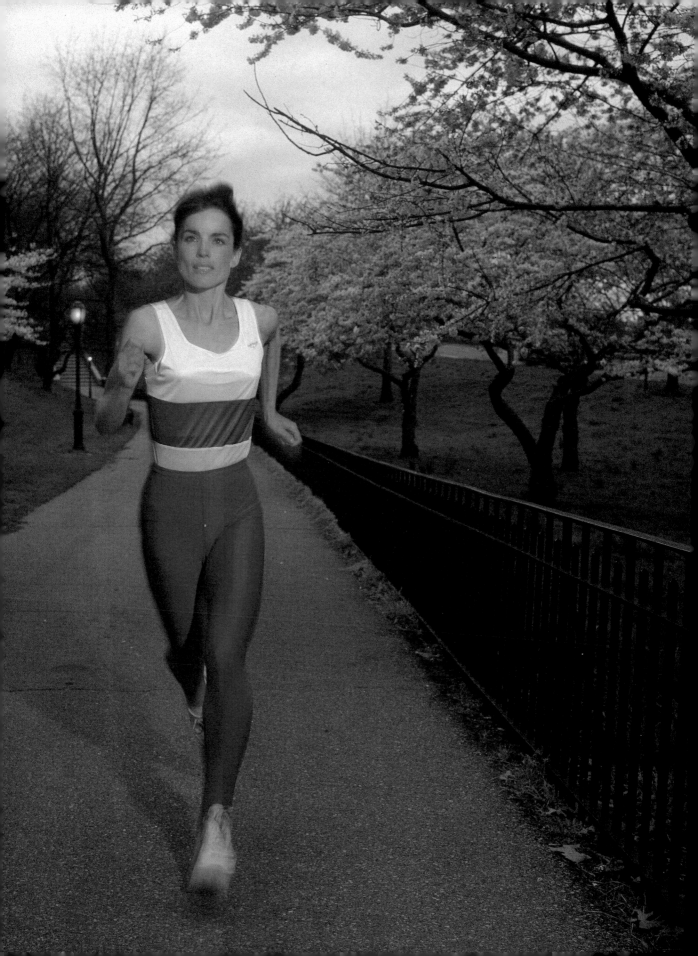

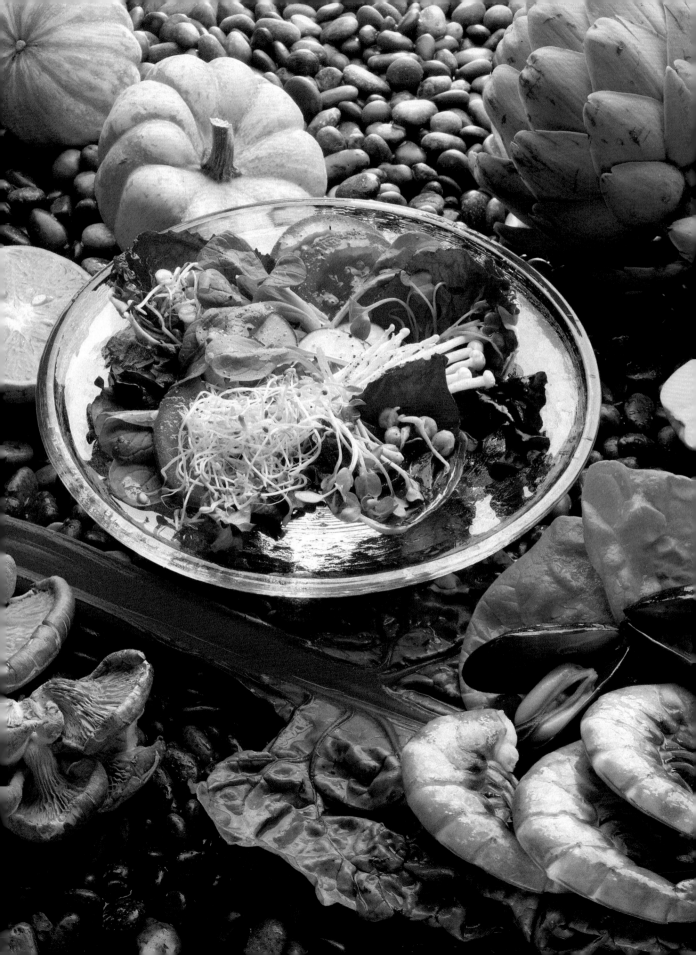

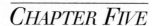
Controlling Cravings

Using nutritious substitutes to discipline your appetite

Most people experience food cravings occasionally. In fact, these cravings can be so intense that even the most disciplined, self-denying person yields to a desire for a particular food, regardless of its nutritional value. Because your preferences for tastes and textures, your emotional state and your environment all have a major impact on what you eat, you may succumb to an urge for food that should be eaten only infrequently, or not at all. Topping the list of foods most often craved are sweets such as candies and cookies, high-fat foods such as ice cream and french fries, and salty foods such as pickles and potato chips. You need not deny your food cravings altogether to maintain a healthy diet; instead, you should find alternate ways to satisfy them.

Although it is hard to pinpoint why cravings occur — despite years of research on which brain mechanism, if any, causes you to crave certain foods, no clear answers have been found — it is not difficult to explain why sweet and salty tastes are appealing. Included in the

The two most often used food additives are sugar and salt, in that order. This list offers healthy, vitamin- and mineral-packed substitutes for popular but overly sweetened or heavily salted foods that people often crave.

SWEET SUBSTITUTES:
Homemade frozen yogurt, sorbet
Baked apple with cinnamon
Frozen ripe banana
Fresh and dried fruit
Natural fruit juices
Cocoa-skim milk shake

LOW- AND NO-SALT SUBSTITUTES:
Spiced low-sodium tomato juice
Bran raisin muffin
Homemade bread
Popcorn with herbs
Unsalted pretzels
Carrot sticks

evidence that establishes the biological basis for eating sweet-tasting foods are studies showing that newborn infants prefer the sweetest liquids they are given. Recent, more controversial research at the Massachusetts Institute of Technology suggests that the hunger for carbohydrate-rich sweets may be correlated with levels of serotonin, a brain chemical that appears to influence mood, appetite and sleep. For some depressed people, an increase of serotonin improves their mood and produces a feeling of satiety. Another possible physiological explanation for a sweet tooth in women involves the menstrual cycle. One study found that women may crave up to 30 percent more carbohydrates during the premenstrual phase of their cycle than at other times.

Sweets are often high in fat and calories, but there are many ways to satisfy your preferences for sweet tastes without jeopardizing a healthy diet. For example, you can train yourself to limit snacks or desserts to just two cookies or, better yet, to fresh fruit. Homemade desserts with little or no sugar added, such as the Pear Tart on page 139 and the Banana Frozen Yogurt on page 140, are better for you than most commercially prepared pies and desserts. If you crave sugary foods such as doughnuts or Danishes for breakfast, replace them with lowfat, unprocessed sweets. Two satisfying examples are the Bran Cereal with Date Milk on page 130 and the Grape and Nut Cereal on page 128.

Unlike the craving for sweets, the desire for highly salted foods is based not on a physiological need but on habit: People who eat a lot of salty foods desensitize themselves to sodium, so food tastes bland to them without it. Salt cravings can become self-perpetuating — the more sodium you eat, the more you want. Fortunately, this pattern can be broken by gradually reducing salt in your diet. One of the problems you will face when trying to restrict your sodium intake is that processed and canned foods with many additives are significantly high in sodium. Eat fresh fruits and vegetables instead of processed ones, restrict salty condiments such as ketchup, mustard and soy sauce, and eliminate salt when cooking by substituting sodium-free spices or herbs. The sodium content of Sweet Potato Shepherd's Pie, on page 136, is only 196 milligrams per serving, as compared with the typical TV dinner, which has 1,000-2,000 milligrams. (The average person needs only 1,000-2,500 milligrams per day.) Too much sodium in the body causes excess water retention and high blood pressure in some people.

People who crave high-fat foods — steak, hamburgers, hot dogs, pastries, ice cream, potato chips — will find that such foods help stave off or satisfy hunger at a considerable cost. Foods that are high in fat slow the passage of food through your stomach, making you feel full, but they contribute to the build-up of fatty deposits in arteries in susceptible people, which can lead to heart attacks, strokes and other problems. These high-calorie foods often include sugar and salt as well. In order to limit your consumption of fatty foods, choose dairy

The Basic Guidelines

For a moderately active adult, the National Institutes of Health recommends a diet that is low in fat, high in carbohydrates and moderate in protein. The institutes' guidelines suggest that no more than 30 percent of your calories come from fat, that 55 to 60 percent come from carbohydrates and that no more than 15 percent come from protein. A gram of fat equals nine calories, while a gram of protein or carbohydrate equals four calories; therefore, if you eat 2,100 calories a day, you should consume approximately 60 grams of fat, 315 grams of carbohydrate and no more than 75 grams of protein daily. If you follow a lowfat/high-carbohydrate diet, your chance of developing heart disease, cancer and other life-threatening diseases may be considerably reduced.

◆ The nutrition charts that accompany each of the lowfat/high-carbohydrate recipes in this book include the number of calories per serving, the number of grams of fat, carbohydrate and protein in a serving, and the percentage of calories derived from each of these nutrients. In addition, the charts provide the amount of calcium, iron and sodium per serving.

◆ Calcium deficiency may be associated with periodontal disease — which attacks the mouth's bones and tissues, including the gums — in both men and women, and with osteoporosis, or bone shrinking and weakening, in the elderly. The deficiency may also contribute to high blood pressure. The recommended daily allowance for calcium is 800 milligrams a day for men and women. Pregnant and lactating women are advised to consume 1,200 milligrams daily; a National Institutes of Health consensus panel recommends that postmenopausal women consume 1,200 to 1,500 milligrams of calcium daily.

◆ Although one way you can reduce your fat intake is to cut your consumption of red meat, you should make sure that you get your necessary iron from other sources. The Food and Nutrition Board of the National Academy of Sciences suggests a minimum of 10 milligrams of iron per day for men and 18 milligrams for women between the ages of 11 and 50.

◆ High sodium intake is associated with high blood pressure. Most adults should restrict sodium intake to between 2,000 and 2,500 milligrams a day, according to the National Academy of Sciences. One way to keep sodium consumption in check is not to add table salt to food.

products made from skim or lowfat milk, which are considerably lower in fat than whole-milk products. A baked potato is preferable to french fries, but do not add generous servings of butter or sour cream. Instead of frying chicken, broil or bake it without the skin.

Perhaps the hardest battles against cravings occur among people on rigid weight-loss regimens. After disciplining themselves to eat only certain foods in fixed quantities, dieters often chafe at all the restrictions. The result can be a food binge. Researchers at the Obesity Clinic at Duke University found that weight-loss diets lack variety in flavor and texture. Their studies showed that compared to their leaner counterparts, overweight people may require more intense taste, aroma and texture from food to satisfy their sensory needs. The recipes that follow, by incorporating a wide variety of foods of different flavors and textures, provide a good foundation for controlling cravings.

Breakfast

GRAPE AND NUT CEREAL

CALORIES per serving	354
58% Carbohydrates	54 g
13% Protein	12 g
29% Fat	12 g
CALCIUM	178 mg
IRON	2 mg
SODIUM	148 mg

Even hearty appetites will be satiated by this generous breakfast. With a combination of toast, cereal, fruit, nuts and yogurt in one bowl, you get filling fiber along with good amounts of calcium and potassium.

1 slice raisin bread
2 tablespoons rolled oats
1/3 cup plain lowfat yogurt
1/4 teaspoon almond extract
Pinch of ground cinnamon
1/2 ounce dried pears

1 teaspoon brown sugar
1/4 cup seedless red grapes
1/4 cup seedless green grapes
2 tablespoons roasted unsalted
   peanuts, coarsely chopped

Preheat the oven to 375° F. Meanwhile, cut the bread into 1/2-inch cubes and spread them and the oats on a foil-lined baking sheet. Bake for 5 to 10 minutes, or until the bread is golden brown; set aside to cool. Stir together the yogurt, almond extract and cinnamon in a cup. Dice the pears; set aside. To serve, place the bread cubes, oats and pears in a cereal bowl and stir to combine. Spoon the yogurt mixture on top and sprinkle it with the sugar. Add the grapes and peanuts, toss gently and serve immediately.

Makes 1 serving

Grape and Nut Cereal

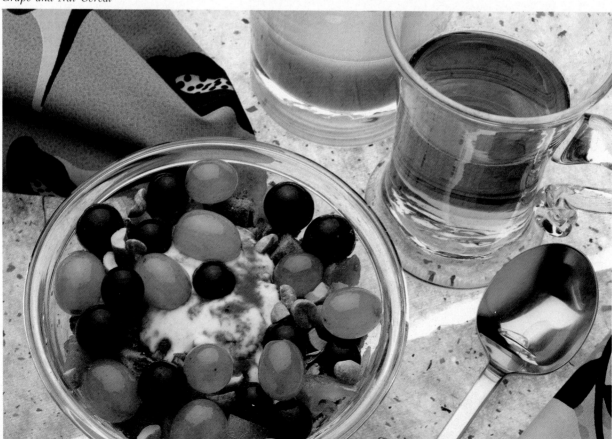

FRENCH TOAST WAFFLES

You may be less tempted by a sugary mid-morning Danish or doughnut if you have this pastry-like dish for breakfast. It has the sweetness of raisins, apple butter and cinnamon, with no refined sugar added.

Vegetable cooking spray
  (optional)
1 egg, beaten
1/2 cup skim milk

1/4 teaspoon cinnamon
4 slices raisin bread
2 tablespoons unsweetened
  apple butter

CALORIES per serving	225
68% Carbohydrates	39 g
15% Protein	9 g
17% Fat	4 g
CALCIUM	131 mg
IRON	2 mg
SODIUM	249 mg

Preheat a nonstick waffle iron. (If your waffle iron does not have a nonstick surface, spray it with cooking spray before heating it. Do not respray the hot iron.) Beat together the egg, milk and cinnamon in a shallow bowl. Dip the bread in the milk mixture, turning it to coat both sides. Place the bread in the waffle iron and cook it for 2 minutes, or until golden brown. Divide the toast waffles among 2 plates and top each serving with 1 tablespoon of apple butter.

Makes 2 servings

BANANA PANCAKES WITH STRAWBERRY SAUCE

It is easy to make your favorite meals more healthful. These pancakes are made without fat, and the fresh berry topping is a high-fiber alternative to bottled pancake syrups, which may be 100 percent sugar.

1 cup fresh strawberries
2 tablespoons plus
  2 teaspoons sugar
1/2 teaspoon cornstarch
1 egg
1/2 cup mashed banana
3/4 cup buttermilk

1/4 cup skim milk
1 1/3 cups unbleached
  all-purpose flour
1 teaspoon baking soda
1/2 teaspoon baking powder
1/2 teaspoon ground cinnamon
Vegetable cooking spray

CALORIES per serving	268
78% Carbohydrates	53 g
13% Protein	8 g
9% Fat	3 g
CALCIUM	123 mg
IRON	2 mg
SODIUM	334 mg

For the sauce, combine the strawberries, 2 teaspoons of sugar and 1 teaspoon of water in a small saucepan, cover and cook over medium-low heat for 10 minutes, or until the strawberries are tender. Increase the heat to medium-high and bring the mixture to a boil. Meanwhile, stir together the cornstarch and 1 teaspoon of water in a cup. Add this mixture to the sauce and cook for 1 minute, or until thickened. Remove the pan from the heat and mash the strawberries with a fork. Cover the pan to keep warm and set aside.

In a small bowl beat together the egg, banana, buttermilk and skim milk; set aside. In a medium-size bowl stir together the flour, the remaining sugar, the baking soda, baking powder and cinnamon, and make a well in the center. Add the egg mixture and stir until well blended.

Spray a large nonstick skillet with cooking spray and heat it over medium-high heat. Pour in four 1/4-cup portions of batter and spread them with a spoon to form 5-inch pancakes. Cook the pancakes for 2 minutes, or until bubbles appear on the tops and the bottoms are golden. Turn the pancakes and cook for another 2 minutes, or until the second side is golden. Transfer the pancakes to a plate and cover them with foil to keep warm. Make 4 more pancakes in the same fashion. Divide the pancakes among 4 plates, spoon the strawberry sauce over them and serve.

Makes 4 servings

SWEET POTATO BISCUITS

CALORIES per biscuit	97
68% Carbohydrates	16 g
7% Protein	2 g
25% Fat	3 g
CALCIUM	46 mg
IRON	1 mg
SODIUM	117 mg

It may be easier to break the habit of reaching for the butter when you eat bread and biscuits if you realize its nutritional cost: A tablespoon of butter has 11 grams of fat and 100 calories. Sweet potato in the dough gives these moist biscuits an unusual flavor that you will enjoy even without butter.

1 cup unbleached all-purpose
  flour, approximately
1 tablespoon brown sugar
2 teaspoons baking powder
Pinch of salt

2 tablespoons plus
  2 teaspoons margarine
1 cup mashed cooked sweet
  potato
1 tablespoon skim milk

Preheat the oven to 450° F. Combine 1 cup of flour, the sugar, baking powder and salt in a food processor. Cut the margarine into small pieces and add it to the dry ingredients while pulsing the machine on and off for 5 to 10 seconds, or until the mixture resembles coarse cornmeal. With the machine running, add the sweet potato and milk, and process for another 5 to 10 seconds, or just until combined. (To mix the dough by hand, stir together the dry ingredients in a medium-size bowl. Cut the margarine into small pieces and then cut it into the dry ingredients with a pastry blender or 2 knives. Add the potato and milk and stir until combined.)

    Remove the dough from the processor or bowl, form it into a ball with your hands and then flatten the dough into a disk. Lightly flour the work surface and a rolling pin, and roll the dough out to a 1/2-inch thickness. Using a 2-inch biscuit cutter, cut 12 biscuits and place them on a baking sheet. Bake the biscuits for 10 minutes, or until they are light golden brown. Serve warm.

Makes 12 biscuits

BRAN CEREAL WITH DATE MILK

CALORIES per serving	339
80% Carbohydrates	81 g
14% Protein	14 g
6% Fat	3 g
CALCIUM	143 mg
IRON	8 mg
SODIUM	533 mg

Adding a fruit-sweetened, lowfat milk mixture makes bran cereal as sweetly satisfying as a heavily sugared breakfast food. You can also serve the milk mixture as a breakfast shake, with some fruit and whole-grain toast or muffins for additional complex carbohydrates and fiber.

1/4 cup fresh strawberries
1/4 cup lowfat cottage
  cheese (1%)
2 ounces pitted dates (5 dates)

3 tablespoons skim milk
1/4 teaspoon vanilla extract
1/2 cup wheat-bran morsels cereal

Wash, hull and halve the strawberries; set aside. Combine the cottage cheese, dates, milk and vanilla in a blender and process for about 10 seconds, or until the mixture is thick and smooth, scraping down the sides of the container with a rubber spatula as necessary. Place the cereal in a bowl and pour the milk mixture over it. Top the cereal with the strawberries and serve immediately.

Makes 1 serving

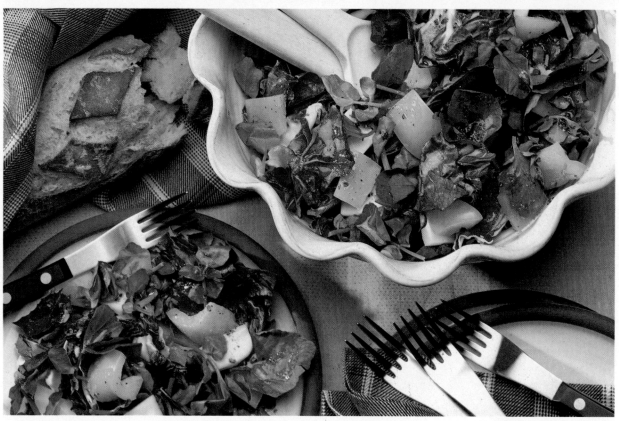

Radicchio-Mozzarella Salad

Lunch

RADICCHIO-MOZZARELLA SALAD

A chef's salad may seem like a good lunch, but the cheese, meat and dressing raise its fat and calorie content greatly. A serving of this salad has just a half-ounce of lowfat cheese and less than a teaspoon of oil.

6 ounces Italian bread
1 tablespoon safflower oil
1/2 cup rice vinegar
2 teaspoons coarse-grain
   Dijon-style mustard
1 garlic clove, crushed and peeled
1/2 teaspoon dried basil
1/4 teaspoon black pepper
Pinch of salt

2 1/2 cups radicchio or red-leaf
   lettuce, torn into bite-size pieces
2 cups watercress, trimmed and
   torn into bite-size pieces
1 medium-size yellow bell pepper,
   cut into 1-inch squares
2 ounces part skim-milk
   mozzarella

CALORIES per serving	205
56% Carbohydrates	29 g
16% Protein	8 g
28% Fat	6 g
CALCIUM	150 mg
IRON	2 mg
SODIUM	438 mg

Preheat the oven to 200° F. Wrap the bread in foil and warm it for 10 minutes. Meanwhile, for the dressing, in a small bowl whisk together the oil, vinegar, mustard, garlic, basil, pepper and salt; set aside. Combine the radicchio, watercress and bell pepper in a salad bowl. Slice the mozzarella into 1-inch squares about 1/4 inch thick and scatter them on top. Whisk the dressing to recombine it, remove the garlic clove and pour the dressing over the salad. Slice the bread and serve it with the tossed salad.   Makes 4 servings

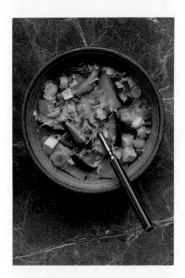

CALORIES per serving	156
55% Carbohydrates	23 g
22% Protein	9 g
23% Fat	4 g
CALCIUM	71 mg
IRON	3 mg
SODIUM	181 mg

HOT AND SOUR SOUP

Ginger, vinegar, tamari, sesame oil and pepper make this Chinese soup flavorful while adding very little sodium.

1 ounce dried shiitake mushrooms	1 teaspoon tamari
2 cups low-sodium chicken stock	1/2 teaspoon Oriental
3/4 cup chopped scallions	sesame oil
1/3 cup sliced bamboo shoots	1/2 teaspoon sugar
1/2 ounce thinly sliced	1/8 teaspoon white pepper
fresh ginger	1 tablespoon plus
2 tablespoons diced tofu	1 teaspoon cornstarch
2 tablespoons rice vinegar	1 egg white

Place the mushrooms in a small bowl, add 2 cups of boiling water and set them aside to soak for 15 minutes.

Reserving the liquid, cut the mushrooms into slivers; set aside. In a large saucepan combine the stock, scallions, bamboo shoots, ginger, tofu, vinegar, tamari, oil, sugar and pepper. Transfer 1/4 cup of the mushroom soaking liquid to a cup and stir in the cornstarch. Add the mushrooms and remaining liquid to the soup and bring it to a boil over medium-high heat. Meanwhile, whisk the egg white in a small bowl. When the soup boils, stir in the cornstarch mixture and the egg white, and cook, stirring, for 1 minute, or until the egg white is opaque. Serve immediately.   Makes 2 servings

BROWN RICE AND VEGETABLE RISOTTO

Risotto's creaminess owes more to the way it is cooked than to added fat. This version contains half the usual amounts of butter and cheese.

2 tablespoons plus	1/2 teaspoon black pepper
1 teaspoon margarine	1 1/2 cups low-sodium
1 cup julienned carrots	chicken stock
1 cup parsnips, sliced	1 1/2 cups chopped scallions
1/8 inch thick	1 cup brown rice
2 cups broccoli florets	1/4 cup grated Parmesan
1/2 teaspoon dried oregano	1/4 cup chopped fresh parsley

CALORIES per serving	332
62% Carbohydrates	53 g
12% Protein	10 g
26% Fat	10 g
CALCIUM	167 mg
IRON	3 mg
SODIUM	229 mg

Melt 1 tablespoon of margarine in a large nonstick skillet over medium-high heat. Add the carrots, parsnips and broccoli, and cook, stirring, for 2 minutes, or until the vegetables are well coated with margarine. Add 1/4 teaspoon of oregano, 1/4 teaspoon of pepper and 1/4 cup of stock, cover and cook for 2 minutes more. Stir in the scallions. Remove the pan from the heat, transfer the vegetables to a bowl and cover it loosely to keep warm.

Melt the remaining margarine in the skillet over medium-high heat. Add the rice, and sauté for 2 minutes. Add 3/4 cup of water, the remaining stock, oregano and pepper. Cover the pan, reduce the heat to medium-low and simmer for 45 minutes, or until the rice is tender and the liquid is almost completely absorbed. Stir in the vegetables, Parmesan and parsley, and cook, stirring, over medium-high heat for 1 minute, or until heated through. Divide the risotto among 4 plates and serve.   Makes 4 servings

BAKED MACARONI AND CHEESE

A serving of this casserole has about half the fat and one third the sodium of a packaged frozen macaroni entrée or mix.

1/4 cup margarine	1 tablespoon coarse-grain
1 cup coarsely chopped onion	Dijon-style mustard
1/3 cup unbleached	1 tablespoon Worcestershire sauce
all-purpose flour	1/4 teaspoon black pepper
1 cup skim milk	10 ounces (2 1/2 cups)
1 cup chopped fresh tomatoes	elbow macaroni
1/4 cup chopped fresh parsley	1/4 cup grated Cheddar cheese

CALORIES per serving	322
59% Carbohydrates	47 g
13% Protein	10 g
28% Fat	10 g
CALCIUM	113 mg
IRON	2 mg
SODIUM	246 mg

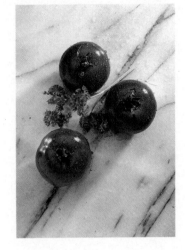

For the sauce, melt the margarine in a medium-size saucepan over medium heat. Add the onion, and cook, stirring, for 5 minutes, or until the onion is translucent. Add the flour and stir until well blended. Slowly add the milk, stirring constantly to prevent lumps from forming. Cook the sauce, stirring frequently, for another 3 to 5 minutes, or until thickened. Stir in the tomatoes, parsley, mustard, Worcestershire sauce and pepper, then remove the pan from the heat, cover and set aside.

Preheat the oven to 350° F. Meanwhile, bring a large pot of water to a boil. Cook the macaroni for 8 minutes, or according to the package directions, until al dente. Drain the macaroni and transfer it to a 1 1/2-quart baking dish. Add the sauce and stir well. Spread the cheese over the macaroni and bake it for 10 to 15 minutes, or until the macaroni is heated through and the cheese is melted. Divide the macaroni among 6 plates and serve.   Makes 6 servings

CHILI-BEAN SLOPPY JOES

These meatless sandwiches, cholesterol-free and rich in iron, are as spicy and filling as Sloppy Joes made with ground beef.

1/2 pound red onions	2 tablespoons tomato paste
3 tablespoons margarine	1 1/2 teaspoons chili powder
1 garlic clove, chopped	1/2 teaspoon brown sugar
One 14-ounce can plum tomatoes	Pinch of salt
2 cups cooked kidney beans, or	Four 2-ounce whole-wheat rolls
canned kidney beans, rinsed	2/3 cup shredded Romaine
and drained	lettuce

Peel and trim the onions. Cut a 1-inch slice from the center of one onion; wrap and set it aside. Coarsely chop the remaining onions. Heat the margarine in a medium-size saucepan over medium heat. Add the chopped onions and garlic, and sauté for 5 minutes, or until the onions are translucent. Add the tomatoes with their liquid, the beans, tomato paste, chili powder, sugar and salt, and bring the mixture to a boil. Cover the pan, reduce the heat to low and simmer the chili for 20 minutes, stirring occasionally.

Ten minutes before serving, preheat the oven to 375° F. Split the rolls, wrap them in foil and heat for 10 minutes. Meanwhile, cut the reserved onion into 4 slices. Place the rolls on 4 plates and top them with the bean mixture. Garnish each sandwich with Romaine and onion, and serve.   Makes 4 servings

CALORIES per serving	380
59% Carbohydrates	59 g
16% Protein	16 g
25% Fat	11 g
CALCIUM	135 mg
IRON	6 mg
SODIUM	672 mg

Dinner
. . . .

SALMON FILET WITH THREE VEGETABLE PUREES

You need not forgo celebratory dinners to eat sensibly, and when you cook a special meal at home you can be sure of the nutritional quality of the dishes you serve. This meal is low in fat and sodium, and high in complex carbohydrates. It is also a good source of calcium, iron, vitamins A and C, and the B vitamins.

CALORIES per serving	465
54% Carbohydrates	63 g
16% Protein	19 g
30% Fat	15 g
CALCIUM	181 mg
IRON	4 mg
SODIUM	412 mg

1/2 pound broccoli
1/2 pound carrots
1/2 pound celery root
2 ounces spinach
1/4 cup margarine
1/3 cup unbleached
  all-purpose flour
1 cup skim milk
1 cup long-grain white rice
Small bunch fresh dill

One 7-ounce salmon filet,
  about 1/2 inch thick
1/8 teaspoon ground nutmeg
1/4 teaspoon salt
2 teaspoons brown sugar
1 garlic clove, peeled
1/4 teaspoon white pepper
2 tablespoons chopped
  fresh parsley

Wash the broccoli, carrots, celery root and spinach. Trim the broccoli and cut it into 1/2-inch pieces. Trim the carrots and cut them into 1-inch pieces. Using a vegetable peeler or a sharp paring knife, trim and peel the celery root; cut it into 1/4-inch-thick slices. Remove any coarse stems from the spinach. Set the vegetables aside.

For the roux, which will form the base of the vegetable purées, melt the margarine in a small saucepan over medium heat. Stir in the flour and mix until blended. Gradually add the milk, whisking constantly until smooth. Cook the roux, stirring constantly, for 1 minute, or until thickened. Transfer the roux to a small bowl, cover and set aside.

Bring 2 cups of water to a boil in a medium-size saucepan over medium-high heat. Stir in the rice. Cover the pan, reduce the heat to medium-low and simmer for 15 minutes, or until the rice is tender and the water is absorbed. When the rice is cooked, remove the pan from the heat and set aside.

While the rice is cooking, bring 1 inch of water to a boil in a saucepan that will accommodate a vegetable steamer. Place the broccoli and spinach in the steamer, cover the pan and cook for 5 minutes, or until the broccoli is tender. Reserving the boiling water in the pan, transfer the broccoli and spinach to a bowl, cover loosely with foil and set aside. Steam the carrots for 5 minutes, or until tender when pierced with a knife; transfer them to a bowl and cover them. Add boiling water to the pan if necessary, then steam the celery root and garlic until tender; transfer them to a bowl, cover and set aside. Reserve the water in the pan for thinning the purées.

Preheat the oven to 400° F. Reserving 4 dill sprigs for garnish, make a bed of half the remaining dill on a large sheet of foil. Place the salmon on top and cover it with the remaining dill. Fold the edges of the foil together to form a packet and bake the salmon for 15 to 20 minutes, or until firm and opaque.

While the salmon is cooking, make the vegetable purées: Purée the broccoli and spinach in a food processor or blender for 10 seconds, or until almost smooth. Add the nutmeg, a pinch of salt and one third of the roux, and process for 5 to 10 seconds more, adding 1 to 2 tablespoons of the hot water from the steamer pan if the purée seems too thick (it should be the consistency of whipped potatoes). Transfer the purée to a bowl and cover it.

Rinse and dry the food processor container. Purée the carrots, adding one third of the roux, the sugar and a pinch of salt; add hot water if necessary. Transfer the purée to a bowl, cover it and set aside. Rinse and dry the container and purée the celery root and garlic with the remaining roux, 1/8 teaspoon of pepper and a pinch of salt; add hot water if necessary. Transfer the purée to a bowl, cover it and set aside.

When the salmon is done, remove it from the oven and set it aside, resealing the packet. Stir the parsley into the rice and divide the rice among 4 plates. Spoon about 1/4 cup of each vegetable purée onto each plate. Open the packet, cut the salmon into 4 pieces and place 1 piece on each plate. Garnish the salmon with the reserved dill sprigs and serve.

Makes 4 servings

Salmon Filet with Three Vegetable Purées

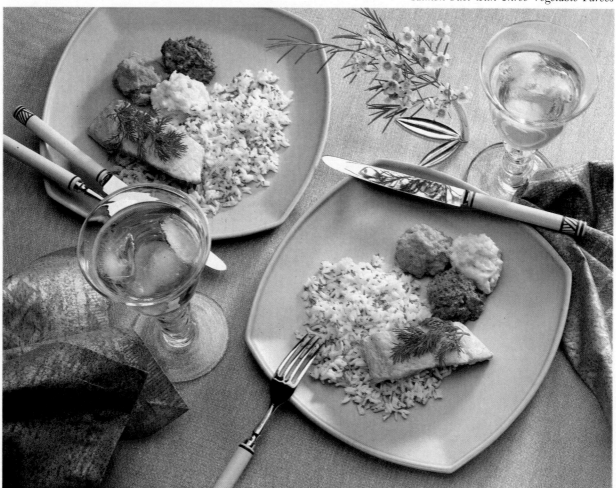

SWEET POTATO SHEPHERD'S PIE

CALORIES per serving	305
56% Carbohydrates	45 g
14% Protein	12 g
30% Fat	10 g
CALCIUM	108 mg
IRON	3 mg
SODIUM	196 mg

Although a mere quarter-pound of lamb is used in this recipe, the meaty flavor pervades the pie's lowfat, high-fiber ingredients as well.

1/4 pound lean ground lamb
1 1/2 cups diced leeks
1 cup chopped onion
2 garlic cloves, chopped
2 tablespoons plus
  2 teaspoons margarine
2 cups diced celery
2 cups sliced zucchini

1 1/2 cups chopped mushrooms
1 cup frozen corn kernels
1/2 cup low-sodium chicken stock
2 teaspoons cornstarch
3/4 teaspoon dried oregano
1 pound sweet potatoes, cooked
2 tablespoons skim milk
Pinch of ground ginger

Heat a large nonstick skillet over medium heat. Add the lamb, breaking it up into small pieces, and cook it for 2 minutes, or until it begins to brown. Add the leeks, onion and garlic, and cook, stirring, for 2 to 3 minutes more, or until the onions and leeks are soft. Add 1 tablespoon of margarine and, when it melts, add the celery, zucchini, mushrooms and corn. Cook, stirring, for 2 minutes, or until the celery softens. Add 1/4 cup of stock and bring the mixture to a boil. Meanwhile, in a small bowl stir together the cornstarch, oregano and remaining stock. Add this mixture to the skillet and cook, stirring constantly, for 1 minute, or until the liquid has thickened; cover and set aside.

Preheat the oven to 400° F. Peel the sweet potatoes, place them in a large bowl and mash them with the milk, ginger and remaining margarine. Turn the lamb mixture into a 9-inch pie plate or a shallow baking dish and spoon the potatoes in a ring on top (or pipe them decoratively with a pastry tube). Bake the pie for 15 to 20 minutes, or until heated through.   Makes 4 servings

MEDALLIONS OF PORK WITH SWEET AND SOUR CABBAGE

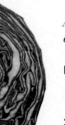

CALORIES per serving	311
57% Carbohydrates	46 g
13% Protein	10 g
30% Fat	11 g
CALCIUM	65 mg
IRON	2 mg
SODIUM	350 mg

A little pork goes a long way in this German-style dish; sautéed apples and cabbage complement its flavor and add complex carbohydrates.

Four 1/4-inch-thick center-cut lean
  loin pork medallions
  (1/4 pound total weight)
2 tablespoons Dijon-style mustard
1 pound small new potatoes
1 medium-size apple
2 tablespoons plus
  2 teaspoons margarine

2 tablespoons brown sugar
4 cups shredded red cabbage
2 tablespoons cider vinegar
1/2 cup unsweetened apple juice
1/4 cup chopped fresh parsley
2 tablespoons unbleached
  all-purpose flour
2 tablespoons sherry

Spread the pork with mustard, wrap it loosely in plastic wrap and set aside. Scrub the potatoes, place them in a medium-size saucepan with cold water to cover and bring to a boil over medium-high heat. Cover the pan, reduce the heat to medium-low and simmer the potatoes for 20 minutes, or until tender.

Meanwhile, wash but do not peel the apple. Core and quarter it and cut it into 1/4-inch-thick slices. Melt 2 teaspoons of margarine in a medium-size skillet over medium-high heat. Add the apple and sauté for 3 minutes. Sprinkle the apple with the sugar and cook for 1 minute, or until the sugar dissolves. Add the cabbage, vinegar and apple juice, bring to a boil and cover the skillet. Reduce the heat to medium and cook for 5 minutes, then uncover the skillet and increase the heat to medium-high. Cook, stirring constantly, for 5 minutes, or until the liquid is almost completely evaporated. Remove the skillet from the heat, stir in 3 tablespoons of parsley, cover and set aside.

Drain and halve the potatoes, return them to the warm pan and toss them with 1 tablespoon of margarine and the remaining parsley; cover and set aside. Melt the remaining margarine in a medium-size nonstick skillet over medium-high heat. Dredge the pork medallions in the flour and cook them for 1 to 2 minutes on each side, or until they are golden-brown all over. Add the sherry and 1 tablespoon of water, and cook for 1 minute more, or until the pan juices thicken. Divide the pork medallions, the potatoes and the cabbage mixture among 4 plates, and serve.   Makes 4 servings

CREOLE CHICKEN STEW WITH BULGUR

Serving bulgur, a whole-grain product, instead of white rice can add to the nutritional value of a stew while providing pleasing variety.

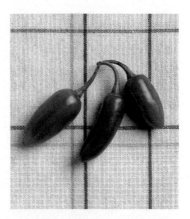

1 cup bulgur	3 cups chopped leeks (1/2 pound)
3 tablespoons plus	2 cups cauliflower florets
1 teaspoon margarine	1 cup red bell pepper,
2 teaspoons arrowroot	cut into 1-inch squares
1/4 pound skinless, boneless	1 cup frozen whole okra
chicken breast, sliced	2 large garlic cloves, peeled
1/4 inch thick	and chopped
1/4 cup white wine	1/2 jalapeño chile, or to taste,
2 tablespoons unbleached	seeded and chopped
all-purpose flour	1/4 teaspoon dried sage
1/2 cup low-sodium chicken stock	1/4 teaspoon dried thyme

CALORIES per serving	375
59% Carbohydrates	57 g
15% Protein	15 g
26% Fat	11 g
CALCIUM	121 mg
IRON	5 mg
SODIUM	165 mg

Bring 2 cups of water to a boil in a medium-size saucepan and stir in the bulgur. Return the water to a boil, cover the pan, reduce the heat to medium-low and simmer for 15 minutes, or until the bulgur is tender and the water is almost completely absorbed. Remove the pan from the heat and set aside.

Melt 1 tablespoon of margarine in a large nonstick skillet over medium-high heat. Meanwhile, spread the arrowroot on a sheet of waxed paper and dredge the chicken in it. Sauté the chicken for 2 minutes, or until it is golden. Add the wine, bring it to a boil and cook the mixture for another minute. Transfer the chicken and cooking liquid to a small bowl, cover it with foil and set aside. Wipe the skillet with a paper towel.

Melt the remaining margarine in the skillet over medium-high heat. Add the flour and stir until blended, then gradually add the stock and 1 cup of water, stirring constantly until smooth. Bring the mixture to a boil and cook for 2 to 3 minutes, or until thickened. Add the leeks, cauliflower, bell pepper, okra, garlic, jalapeño, sage and thyme, and return the mixture to a boil. Cover the pan, reduce the heat to medium-low and simmer for 10 minutes, or until the vegetables are just tender. Bring the stew to a full boil, add the chicken and cooking liquid, and cook, stirring, for 1 minute, or until heated through. Divide the bulgur among 4 plates and spoon the stew on top.   Makes 4 servings

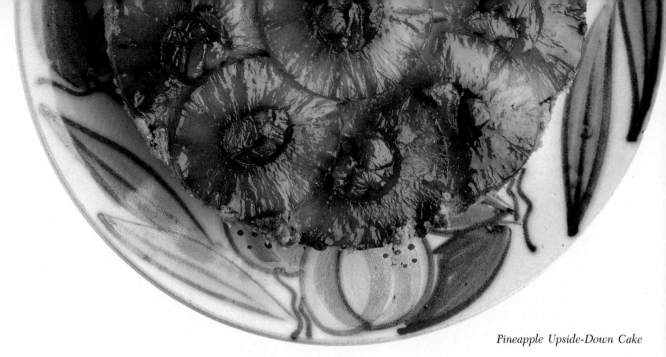

Pineapple Upside-Down Cake

Desserts

PINEAPPLE UPSIDE-DOWN CAKE

Foods that offer a variety of flavors and textures — like this dessert, with its crisp crust, juicy topping and smooth cake — are especially satisfying, so a small portion suffices.

CALORIES per serving	246
76% Carbohydrates	48 g
5% Protein	3 g
19% Fat	6 g
CALCIUM	61 mg
IRON	2 mg
SODIUM	174 mg

1/4 cup plus 2 teaspoons
  margarine
10 tablespoons brown sugar
One 20-ounce can juice-packed
  pineapple slices, drained,
   1 cup of juice reserved
1/3 cup coarsely chopped
  dried apricots

1 1/2 cups unbleached
  all-purpose flour
1 1/4 teaspoons baking powder
1/2 teaspoon baking soda
Pinch of salt
1 egg
1 cup dark raisins

Grease an 8-inch cake pan with 2 teaspoons of margarine and sprinkle 2 tablespoons of sugar in the bottom. Arrange the pineapple slices in the pan, overlapping them slightly, and fill the hole in each slice with apricots.

Preheat the oven to 350° F. In a small bowl stir together the flour, baking powder, baking soda and salt; set aside. In a medium-size bowl, using an electric mixer, cream together the margarine and remaining sugar. Add the egg, and beat until well blended. Beat in the dry ingredients and pineapple juice alternately, in 3 parts each. Stir in the raisins and pour the batter into the pan. Gently tap the pan on the countertop to settle the batter, then bake for 1 hour, or until the cake is golden brown on top and pulls away from the sides of the pan. Let the cake cool on a rack for 5 minutes. Run a knife around the edge of the pan to loosen the cake, then place a platter over the pan and invert it. Leave the pan on the cake for a moment, tap it gently, then carefully lift the pan to turn out the cake. Makes 10 servings

PEAR TART

A low-calorie dessert at dinner can help you resist late-night snacks.

CALORIES per serving	202
63% Carbohydrates	32 g
7% Protein	3 g
30% Fat	7 g
CALCIUM	14 mg
IRON	1 mg
SODIUM	99 mg

1 1/4 cups unbleached
  all-purpose flour
7 tablespoons sugar
Pinch of salt

1/4 cup margarine, well chilled
2 ripe Comice pears
1 egg plus 1 egg white
1 teaspoon almond extract

In a medium-size bowl stir together 1 cup of flour, 2 tablespoons of sugar and the salt. Using a pastry blender or 2 knives, cut in the margarine until the mixture resembles cornmeal. Add 2 to 3 tablespoons of cold water and stir until the mixture forms a dough. Knead the dough for 1 minute, then form it into a ball. Flatten it into a disk, wrap and refrigerate for 20 minutes.

Dust the work surface and a rolling pin with 1 tablespoon of flour. Roll out the dough to a 12-inch circle and transfer it to a 9-inch tart pan with a removable bottom. Gently press the dough into the pan, then trim the edges; set aside.

Preheat the oven to 425° F. Peel, core and quarter the pears and slice them 1/4 inch thick; set aside. In a small bowl beat together the whole egg, egg white, almond extract, 2 tablespoons of sugar and the remaining flour. Arrange the pears in the crust, pour the egg mixture over them and bake the tart for 10 minutes. Reduce the heat to 350° F; turn the pan if the crust is not browning evenly. Sprinkle the tart with the remaining sugar and bake for 25 minutes more, or until the custard is set and the crust is golden brown. (Any liquid remaining on top of the custard will be absorbed as the tart cools.) Let the tart cool on a rack for 5 minutes and serve warm. Makes 8 servings

CAROB FUDGE CAKE

A slice of this dense, chocolaty-tasting cake — even with a dollop of creamy topping — has less than half the fat and sugar of cake made from a mix.

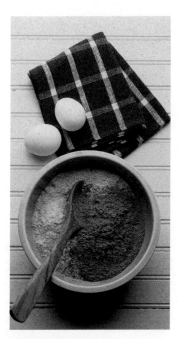

Vegetable cooking spray
1 1/2 cups unbleached
  all-purpose flour, approximately
1/2 cup carob powder
1 teaspoon baking powder
1 teaspoon baking soda

2 tablespoons margarine
2/3 cup sugar
2 eggs
1 teaspoon vanilla extract
1 1/2 cups buttermilk
1/2 cup nonbutterfat sour dressing

Preheat the oven to 350° F. Spray an 8-inch baking pan with cooking spray and dust it lightly with flour; set aside. In a small bowl stir together 1 1/2 cups of flour, the carob powder, baking powder and baking soda; set aside. In a medium-size bowl cream together the margarine and sugar. Beat in the eggs one at a time. Add the vanilla and half the buttermilk, then stir in half the dry ingredients. Add the remaining buttermilk and beat until blended, then beat in the remaining dry ingredients. Pour the batter into the pan and gently tap it to level the batter. Bake for 35 minutes, or until the cake begins to pull away from the sides of the pan and a toothpick inserted into the center comes out clean and dry. Let the cake cool on a rack for 5 minutes, then run a knife around the edge to loosen it and turn it out. Cut the cake into 10 wedges and top each portion with a dollop of sour dressing. Makes 10 servings

CALORIES per serving	206
63% Carbohydrates	33 g
10% Protein	5 g
27% Fat	6 g
CALCIUM	93 mg
IRON	1 mg
SODIUM	221 mg

Snacks and Beverages

BANANA FROZEN YOGURT

*Extra calcium and potassium are nutritional bonuses when you make
your own frozen dessert with lowfat yogurt and fresh fruit.*

4 medium-size bananas	1/2 teaspoon coconut extract
1/2 cup sugar	3 cups plain lowfat yogurt

Peel 2 bananas, combine them with the sugar and coconut extract in a food
processor, and process until puréed. Add the yogurt, and process for 5 to 10
seconds, or until blended. Or mash the bananas with a fork in a medium-size
bowl, add the sugar and extract, then stir in the yogurt. Turn the mixture into
the container of an ice cream maker and freeze it according to the manufac-
turer's instructions until thick and creamy. If not serving the frozen yogurt
immediately, cover the container tightly and place it in the freezer.

Peel and slice the remaining bananas. If necessary, let the frozen yogurt
soften at room temperature for 5 minutes. Divide the yogurt and the banana
slices among 8 dessert dishes, and serve.   Makes 8 servings

CALORIES per serving	161
79% Carbohydrates	32 g
12% Protein	5 g
9% Fat	2 g
CALCIUM	159 mg
IRON	.2 mg
SODIUM	60 mg

Banana Frozen Yogurt

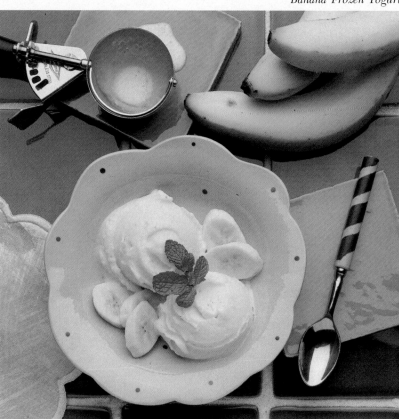

PEAR NECTAR

You can satisfy a sugar craving with sweets that are also nutritious: This spicy fruit nectar is a better choice than a heavily sugared soft drink. Enjoy this beverage over ice as a refreshing reward after exercise, or drink it hot as a relaxing break during an active day.

1 ripe Comice pear
1/2 cup unsweetened apple juice
1/4 teaspoon maple syrup

Pinch of ground ginger
1 cinnamon stick (optional)

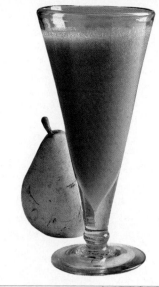

Peel, core and coarsely dice the pear; you should have about 1 cup. Place the pear, apple juice, maple syrup and ginger in a small saucepan and bring it to a boil over medium-high heat. Cover the pan, reduce the heat to medium-low and simmer the mixture for 5 minutes, or until the pear is tender. Transfer the mixture to a food processor or blender and process it for 10 seconds, or until smoothly puréed. If the purée seems too thick, add a little hot water. Serve the pear nectar hot, with a cinnamon stick, if desired, or refrigerate it until well chilled and serve it cold, over ice if desired.   Makes 1 serving

CALORIES per serving	161
94% Carbohydrates	41 g
2% Protein	1 g
4% Fat	1 g
CALCIUM	29 mg
IRON	1 mg
SODIUM	4 mg

BABAGANOUSH

Keeping a lowfat spread like this eggplant purée on hand helps you avoid the temptation of fatty sour cream or cream cheese dips. Add some crisp vegetable sticks or whole-wheat pita triangles as dippers for a nutritious snack.

1 3/4 pounds eggplant
1 garlic clove
1 tablespoon plus
  1 teaspoon margarine
3 tablespoons unbleached
  all-purpose flour
3/4 cup skim milk

1/4 cup lowfat cottage
  cheese (1%)
2 tablespoons chopped
  fresh parsley
1 tablespoon lemon juice
1/2 teaspoon salt

Preheat the broiler. Stem and halve the eggplant and place the halves cut side down on a foil-lined baking sheet. Broil the eggplant 6 inches from the heat for 15 minutes, or until the skin is well charred. Reduce the oven temperature to 375° F. (Transfer the eggplant from the broiler to the oven if using a separate broiler.) Place the unpeeled garlic on the baking sheet. Bake the eggplant and garlic for 15 minutes; remove them from the oven and set aside to cool. Melt the margarine in a small saucepan over medium heat. Peel and mash the garlic, add it to the pan and cook for 2 minutes. Whisk in the flour and continue whisking until smooth, then gradually add the milk, whisking constantly until the mixture forms a smooth, thick sauce. Remove the pan from the heat and set aside.

   Place the cottage cheese in a food processor or blender and process it for 5 to 10 seconds, or until smooth. Add the garlic sauce and process the mixture for 5 seconds more. Scoop the eggplant flesh into the processor, add the parsley, lemon juice and salt, and process for another 5 seconds, or just until combined. Transfer the babaganoush to a bowl and serve immediately, or cover and refrigerate it until well chilled.   Makes 6 servings

CALORIES per serving	84
54% Carbohydrates	12 g
18% Protein	4 g
28% Fat	3 g
CALCIUM	88 mg
IRON	1 mg
SODIUM	272 mg

PROP CREDITS

Cover: tank top–Naturalife, New York City, shorts–Athletic Style, New York City, sneakers–Nautilus Athletic Footwear, Inc., Greenville, S.C., location courtesy of Herricks High School, New Hyde Park, N.Y.; page 6: T-shirt and shorts–Athletic Style, New York City, sneakers–Nautilus Athletic Footwear, Inc., Greenville, S.C., towel–Martex, New York City, location courtesy of Jerome S. Coles Sports and Recreation Center, New York University, New York City; page 22: leotard–Dance France, LTD., Santa Monica, Calif.; pages 26-33: tank top and sweat pants–Athletic Style, New York City; pages 28-31: towel–Martex, New York City; pages 34-51: leotard and tights–Athletic Style, New York City, mat–AMF American, Jefferson, Iowa; pages 51-55: towel–Martex, New York City; pages 52-63: tank top and sweat pants–Athletic Style, New York City, mat–AMF American, Jefferson, Iowa; page 64: sweat pants–Athletic Style, New York City; pages 68-83: leotard–Marika, courtesy of The Weekend Exercise Co., San Diego, Calif., sweat pants–The Gap, San Francisco, Calif.; pages 84-89: sweat pants–Athletic Style, New York City; pages 94-105: tank tops and sweat pants–Athletic Style, New York City; page 106: diving briefs–The Finals, Port Jervis, N.Y., location courtesy of Jerome S. Coles Sports and Recreation Center, New York University, New York City; page 110: top–Nike, Inc., Beaverton, Ore., sneakers–Nautilus Athletic Footwear, Inc., Greenville, S.C.; pages 112-113: bathing suit–The Finals, Port Jervis, N.Y., location courtesy of Jerome S. Coles Sports and Recreation Center, New York University, New York City, towel–Martex, New York City; page 114: T-shirt–Athletic Style, New York City, cycling shorts–The Finals, Port Jervis, N.Y., touring shoes–Nike, Inc., Beaverton, Ore.; page 116: T-shirt and shorts–Athletic Style, New York City, sneakers–Nautilus Athletic Footwear, Inc., Greenville, S.C., basketball–Cutler-Owens, Inc., New York City, location courtesy of Jerome S. Coles Sports and Recreation Center, New York University, New York City; pages 118-119: location courtesy of Herricks High School, New Hyde Park, N.Y.; page 120: tank top–Athletic Style, New York City; page 122: tank top–The Finals, Port Jervis, N.Y., sneakers–Nike, Inc., Beaverton, Ore.; page 128: glass, mug, bowl and spoon–Simon Pearce, New York City, napkins–Frank McIntosh at Henri Bendel, New York City; page 131: salad bowl, plates and flatware–Simon Pearce, New York City, salad servers–Pottery Barn, New York City, napkins–Frank McIntosh at Henri Bendel, New York City; page 132: bowl–Simon Pearce, New York City, spoon–Thaxton & Co., New York City; page 135: plates–Frank McIntosh at Henri Bendel, New York City, flatware–Simon Pearce, New York City; page 138: plate–Frank McIntosh at Henri Bendel, New York City; page 140: spoon–Thaxton & Co., New York City, napkin–Frank McIntosh at Henri Bendel, New York City, tiles–Country Floors, New York City; page 141: glass–Gear, New York City.

ACKNOWLEDGMENTS

All cosmetics and grooming products supplied by Clinique Labs, Inc., New York City

Nutrition analysis provided by Hill Nutrition Associates, Fayetteville, N.Y.

Off-camera warm-up equipment: rowing machine supplied by Precor USA, Redmond, Wash.; Tunturi stationary bicycle supplied by Amerec Corp., Bellevue, Wash.

Washing machine and dryer supplied by White-Westinghouse, Columbus, Ohio

Index prepared by Ian Tucker

Production by Giga Communications

ILLUSTRATION CREDITS

Illustration, page 9: David Flaherty; all other charts and illustrations: Brian Sisco

INDEX

motivation, 12, 20
for non-athletes, 14
performance consistency and, 8
program of, *see* mental training
program
self-confidence and, 13
stress and, *see* stress
techniques of, *see* concentration;
relaxation; visualization
mental training program, 16-21
goal setting, 20-21
motivation, 20
self-assessment, 16-17
see also concentration; relaxation;
visualization
monoamines, 12-13
motivation, 12, 20, 107
Moving Concentration sequence, 80-83
Moving Meditation sequence, 72-79
muscles
influence of mind on, 19
relaxation of, *see* relaxation

Narrow-external concentration, 10
narrow-internal concentration, 10
neurotransmitters, 12-13

Optimal arousal, zone of, 11
osteoporosis, 127
oxygen consumption, 24

Parasympathetic nervous system, 9
positive goals, 21
positive thinking, 12, 13
previewing, 110-111
progressive relaxation, 25
protein
amounts in recipe dishes, 128-141
recommended intake of, 127

Recipes
beverage, 141
breakfast, 128-130
dessert, 138-139

dinner, 134-137
lunch, 131-133
snack, 140, 141
relaxation, 11, 23-63
body scan, 25
combined with visualization, 15, 18
deep breathing, *see* deep breathing
meditation, *see* meditation
progressive, 25
relaxation response, 25
for sports, 112-113
Yoga, *see* Yoga
relaxation response, 25
rituals, 116-117
rolls
back, 92-93
front, 90-91
rotational throw, 98-99

Salted foods, controlling cravings for,
126
selective attention, *see* concentration
self-confidence, 13
serotonin, 126
shifting focus, 122-123
short-term vs. long-term goals, 21
Shoulder Stand position, 54-55
snack recipes, 140, 141
sodium
amounts in recipe dishes, 128-141
controlling cravings for, 126
recommended intake of, 127
Spinal Twist position, 46-47
sports, *see* focusing for sports
Stork position, 60-61
stress
control of, 9, 24
need for, 11
neurotransmitters and, 12-13
see also anxiety
stretching, 112
see also Yoga
Sumo, 67
Sun Salutation position, 38-45

sweet foods, controlling cravings for,
126
sword sequence, 84-89
sympathetic nervous system, 9, 23-24

Table position, 41, 44
Tae kwon do, 67
task-relevant and task-irrelevant cues,
109
Tibetan meditative position, 30-31

Visualization, 13-14, 18
combined with relaxation, 15, 18
defined, 14
drills, 19
previewing, 110-111
process of, 18
for sports, 110-111, 118-119

Warm-ups, Yoga, 32-35
Warrior position, 52-53
winning, focus on mastery vs.,
12, 16

Yoga, 32-63
asanas, 24, 32, 36
Dove position, 50-51
Downward-Facing Dog position,
36-37
Eagle position, 58-59
Fish position, 56-57
Headstand position, 62-63
Head to Knee position, 48-49
physical fitness benefits of, 24
psychological effects of, 24
Shoulder Stand position, 54-55
Spinal Twist position, 46-47
sports and, 112
Stork position, 60-61
Sun Salutation position, 38-45
warm-ups, 32-35
Warrior position, 52-53

Zen meditation, 24, 25, 30